570

ALLEN COUNTY PUBLIC LIBRARY

FORT WAYNE, INDIANA 46802

You may return this book to any agency, branch,
or bookmobile of the Allen County Public Library.

DEMCO

New Choices:

The Latest Options in Treating Breast Cancer

New Choices:

The Latest Options in Treating Breast Cancer

Mark Rubinstein, M.D.
Dennis P. Cirillo, M.D.

· · · ·

DODD, MEAD & COMPANY
NEW YORK

To Our Patients

No part of this book may be reproduced in any form
without permission in writing from the publisher.
Published by Dodd, Mead & Company, Inc.
79 Madison Avenue, New York, N.Y. 10016
Distributed in Canada by
McClelland and Stewart Limited, Toronto
Manufactured in the United States of America
First Edition

Library of Congress Cataloging in Publication Data

Rubinstein, Mark, 1942–
   New choices.

   Includes index.
   1. Breast—Cancer—Treatment.   I. Cirillo, Dennis P.
II. Title.
RC280.B8R83   1985   616.99′44906   84-24726
ISBN 0-396-08552-0

Contents

Foreword by Richard C. Simons, M.D.   vii

Introduction   ix

One ❧ What Is Breast Cancer?   1

Two ❧ Who Develops Breast Cancer?   10

Three ❧ Detecting a Lump   26

Four ❧ I've Found a Lump—What Do I Do?   49

Five ❧ The Meanings of Breast Cancer   67

Six ❧ It's Cancer—What Next?   86

Seven ❧ Systemic Therapies for Breast Cancer   114

Eight ❧ Your Treatment: How to Deal with It   120

Nine ❧ How Has My Life Changed?   139

Ten ❧ Breast Reconstruction   165

Eleven ❧ Life Beyond Breast Cancer   190

Twelve ❧ The Future   199

Index   207

Foreword

New Choices: The Latest Options in Treating Breast Cancer
is a remarkable accomplishment. Written jointly by a psychiatrist (Mark Rubinstein, M.D.) and a surgeon (Dennis P. Cirillo, M.D.), this book is uniquely informative not only to
laypersons of all backgrounds but to health care professionals and medical specialists as well. The authors have taken
a complex, emotionally charged subject and have presented
it in a clear, straightforward manner that offers both truth
and hope to all of us. The causes of breast cancer, the diagnosis, the prognosis, the prevention, the psychological impact
on patients and their loved ones, the multiple therapeutic
and reconstructive approaches now available—all these aspects and many more are discussed through the use of poi-
gnant case histories and vivid question-answer formats. Drs.
Rubinstein and Cirillo have indeed been faithful to their
closing message: ". . . every woman must be responsible

for her health and be willing to play an active role in learning her treatment choices and maintaining her own well-being."

Richard C. Simons, M.D.
Professor of Psychiatry
University of Colorado School
of Medicine
Denver, Colorado

Introduction

Each year, 3 million women consult a physician because of a breast lump that turns out to be benign. In a recent survey conducted by the Opinion Research Corporation of Princeton, New Jersey, three-quarters of all women interviewed ranked the fear of developing breast cancer as their most important health concern. Yet, despite the fear this disease evokes, most women know very little about it.

Breast cancer is an emotional and physical crisis in the life of any woman and her family. Like any crisis, it requires a clear head and rational approach if it is going to be solved. Over time we have developed the conviction that our patients and the millions of people like them could be helped by a book which would demystify breast cancer and make it less frightening. Though there are books about this topic, none focus on breast cancer in all its emotional and physical dimensions. As a psychiatrist and a surgeon, we have done exactly that.

This book is for *every woman,* whether you are now a patient or not! Based on our work (separately and together) with patients, it is a step-by-step guide to dealing with breast cancer. It is an accurate and complete guide for everything you need to know about this disease: its earliest diagnosis, its treatment, its long-term follow-up, and guidelines for physical and emotional rehabilitation.

Reading this book will arm you with the latest information. You will know how cancer develops. You will learn if you are a high-risk candidate and how to deal with your risk. You will learn the telltale signs and symptoms of breast cancer and how to recognize them—early! You will learn the step-by-step diagnostic plan of action needed to have a breast lump medically investigated. You will know the latest options for treating breast cancer. You will learn that today, no one need go through life with only one breast. We have also included in several chapters a section called "Frequently Asked Questions," providing answers to concerns our patients have often voiced.

In-depth personal interviews with patients and their families are included. Here, women who have dealt with breast cancer reveal their most intimate thoughts and feelings about it: how they struggled with fear of recurrence; with feelings of depression; and with concerns about their partners, their sexual lives, the future, and their relationships with children, friends, and coworkers. You will see how other people—women and men—successfully coped with breast cancer. Each made changes and adapted to new realities and challenges. For many, the experience of breast cancer—as frightening as it was—led to a greater capacity for intimacy and personal growth and to a discovery of new strengths and resources they never knew they possessed.

Today, with better cancer detection methods and a variety of treatment options, including less disfiguring surgery, radiation, chemotherapy, and new reconstructive techniques, the outlook is better than ever before. Knowing all this will make you less afraid of breast cancer. Being less afraid will make you more willing to *self-examine* and *go for treatment early* if a lump is discovered. Then, the chance of cure is greatest. It will dramatically improve your chances of living a normal life even if you *do* become a patient.

Knowing all this can change your life and the lives of those who love you. That is why we wrote this book.

Mark Rubinstein, M.D.
Dennis P. Cirillo, M.D.

ONE

What Is
Breast Cancer?

To understand breast cancer and how it develops, there are certain facts one should know about cells and how they work.

The Cell

Every organ, including the breast, is composed of millions of basic structural units called cells. A *cell* is a microscopic bit of protoplasm that, along with other cells of an organ (the breast, liver, the heart) has two primary purposes:

First, the cell produces energy so it can work as part of an organ. Each cell takes part in the maintenance, nutrition, and repair of the organ so the body may function normally.

Second, each cell must reproduce itself. This is necessary because all organs require replacement or repair of their tissues owing to ordinary wear and tear. It is this special function of cells—their capacity to reproduce themselves—which is pathologically altered in cancer.

Cell Division

All cells reproduce by first duplicating their chromosomes, which contain their genetic material, and by then dividing in half to form two daughter cells. This is called *mitosis*. In this process, cells operate according to a biological "clock" and reproduce at different rates of speed. For example, normal blood and skin cells divide and subdivide very quickly because they ordinarily wear out quickly and must be rapidly replaced. Normal liver cells, on the other hand, have a much longer life span and reproduce themselves slowly.

How Cancer Develops

Normally, cells throughout the body reproduce themselves in an orderly manner so that growth occurs, worn out tissues are replaced, and injuries are repaired. This is not the case with cancer cells. Cancer is a disease characterized by uncontrolled rapid growth and the spread of abnormal cells. This results in a mass, or tumor, within the affected organ. This abnormally sped-up reproduction of cells is the basic problem in all cancers.

Although no one knows why and how cancer cells form, several theories are being investigated. Many researchers think cancer is basically genetic; that it is "passed on" from parent to child within the chromosomes of each cell. Certain types of cancer do tend to run in families, and breast cancer is one of them. This theory contends that when various environmental factors are present, cancer will eventually develop.

Other researchers emphasize the possibility that certain cancers are caused by a mutation, a pathological change of some kind, within the cell's reproductive apparatus. When such a mutation occurs, a cancer may appear.

Evidence is accumulating that cancer can be triggered by certain environmental factors. These may include certain chemicals (Agent Orange, nitrites) certain viruses, radiation (overexposure to x-rays or nuclear radiation), or even the ultraviolet rays of the sun. The precise mechanism or mechanisms of these abnormal changes is unknown, but it is clear that certain cellular changes result in the proliferation of abnormal cells. These cells can then overgrow themselves and invade nearby tissues or even spread to other organs.

About Tumors

A *tumor,* by definition, is a swelling in tissue. It can be caused by infection, by inflammation, or by cell reproduction, as in cancer. Here, we are concerned with tumors caused by the abnormally rapid division of cells into a cancerous mass.

A tumor may be benign or malignant. *Benign* tumors are usually harmless, although some may interfere with an organ's function because of their location. For instance, a benign brain tumor may cause trouble because it is contained within the skull, where there is no room for expansion. It can then press on other brain structures and surgery may be required. However, benign tumors do not invade neighboring tissues and do not spread to other parts of the body. Therefore, benign masses rarely threaten life.

Malignant tumors (*malignant* literally means "evil or malicious") are caused by cellular changes that result in rapidly proliferating cancer tissue. Over the course of time they may invade and destroy normal tissue either by encroaching into nearby organs or by spreading widely throughout the body. This is called a *metastasis.* Malignant cancer cells may break away (or metastasize) from the original tumor and spread to other parts of the body, where they can lodge and form new, or *secondary,* cancers. If a breast cancer metastasizes to the liver, a pathologist can usually recognize these secondary cancer cells within the liver as *breast* cancer cells. Such abnormal, rapidly proliferating breast tissue cells may expand and exert their influence in the liver. This process of metastasis and growth may occur in many organs and, if unchecked, eventually causes death.

The Anatomy of the Breast

Understanding something about the anatomy of the breast will help explain how breast cancer may spread and why it is treated the way it is.

The normal breast is composed of several different tissues. Just beneath the skin is a layer of subcutaneous fat, then there is fascia, a membranelike covering overlying the breast tissue and also separating it from the underlying muscles of the chest wall. Two muscles lie just beneath the breast tissue: the pectoralis major and the pectoralis minor. Milk glands, located throughout the breast tissue, connect to a system of ducts to form lobules, which radiate out from the nipple (see Figure 1).

The Lymphatic System

The lymphatic system is located throughout the body. Its fluid carries waste-removing cells that form an integral part of the immune system and protect the body from disease. This intricate surveillance and defense system can detect and destroy invading foreign matter such as bacteria, viruses, or cancer cells.

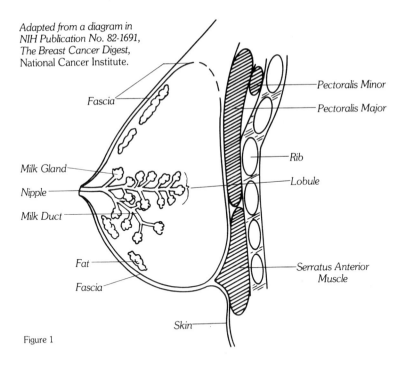

Adapted from a diagram in
NIH Publication No. 82-1691,
The Breast Cancer Digest,
National Cancer Institute.

Pectoralis Minor

Pectoralis Major

Fascia

Rib

Milk Gland

Lobule

Nipple

Milk Duct

Fat

Serratus Anterior
Muscle

Fascia

Skin

Figure 1

Throughout the lymphatic ducts there are defensive way stations or outposts called lymph nodes. These clusters of tissue manufacture the white blood cells, which trap and attack any invading cells reaching them. If effective, this prevents the cancer cells from spreading throughout the lymphatic system and reaching other parts of the body. But the nodes may not stop all the cancer cells. In fact, they may sometimes be overwhelmed, and the lymph nodes themselves may be replaced by the cancer cells. If cancer cells are present in the lymph nodes, the nodes are said to be "positive" for cancer when they are examined by a surgeon.

Tumors of the outer half of the breast, those formed between the nipple and the armpit, usually drain into the axillary lymph nodes for that breast. (*Axilla* means "armpit.") Tumors of the inner half of the breast drain into the internal mammary chain of lymph nodes located alongside the ste·

num, or breast bone. They also drain into the lymph nodes located beneath the muscle tissue of the chest wall (see Figure 2).

Changes in Breast Tissue

Before breast cancer can develop, at some point normal breast tissue cells change into cancerous cells. No one is certain precisely how or when this happens. But all women have certain cyclic changes in their breast tissue until they reach menopause.

At puberty, when a girl begins menstruating, her breasts prepare themselves for the possibility of pregnancy and of providing milk. The breast tissue cells of all menstruating women undergo monthly changes in response to varying hormonal influences during the menstrual cycle. With these

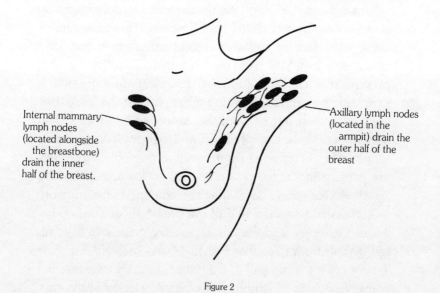

Internal mammary lymph nodes (located alongside the breastbone) drain the inner half of the breast.

Axillary lymph nodes (located in the armpit) drain the outer half of the breast

Figure 2

monthly changes, which include the tissue's swelling, engorging, and then shrinking, there may sometimes be a blockage of the milk ducts. This may cause small cysts to form or other slight changes in the breast tissue. Physicians have long recognized these benign changes and have grouped them together under the name *fibrocystic disease of the breast.* Virtually half of all women have some form of this condition, which accounts for 80 percent of all breast lumps. There are several types of cellular change that occur within this broad group. In an effort to detect breast cancer earlier, researchers have tried to determine if some of these cellular changes may herald the later development of breast cancer.

So far, it is very difficult to determine this, and the point at which cells are about to possibly become malignant is still open to debate. In many women, these benign cellular changes never progress to cancer and, in fact, may even revert back to normal-looking cells. Breast tissue, then, is subject to many variables, and any tissue frequently upset or changed by physiological influences, no matter how normal, has a greater potential for problems. An analogy would be a machine with many moving parts; such a machine would have a greater chance of malfunctioning than another with fewer parts and less complexity.

A Breast Cancer Develops

At some point, breast cells may change and become cancerous. They may then begin rapidly reproducing and form a tumor. By the time a breast lump can be felt it is at least 1 centimeter in size, or about the size of a pea. Medical studies have been done to determine how quickly cancer cells divide and form a tumor. The dividing time for abnormal breast cells can be anywhere from 23 to 209 days. This is the time it takes for the cell to split in half and duplicate itself once. This means that a cancerous tumor could be present in the breast from 2 to 17 years before it is large enough to be felt by the human hand.

During all this time, cancer cells from the tumor may have been shed into the lymphatic system that drains the breast (see Figure 2). Or they may have gone into the blood stream to circulate throughout the body, where they can lodge and form secondary tumors. This process of uncontrolled cell division does not go unrecognized by the body. The lymphatic system plays a crucial role in determining if these cells continue to divide and spread or if they are recognized and killed in the lymph nodes. The capacity to resist the invading cancer cells varies from one person to another and the success of the body's defenses depends also on how fast or slowly the invading cancer cells multiply.

Cancer can form anywhere in the breast, but it is usually found within the glandular tissue, most often within the milk ducts. These cancers may be invasive or noninvasive.

Sometimes a single cancer tumor may be made up of several different types of cells (milk gland and milk duct tissue, along with connective tissue). Each may have a different rate of growth and a different potential to metastasize throughout the body. An *in situ* cancer is one which is confined to its site of origin. It has not invaded the surrounding tissues. But this kind of cancer may eventually become invasive and may metastasize. There is no way to predict which tumor will remain confined to its original site or which will eventually become invasive.

In summary, there are different types of tumors arising from different parts of the breast. There are varying rates of growth in different tumors. There may even be different rates of growth for the same kind of tumor in one patient as compared to another. There are varying potentials for a particular cancer to remain confined to its site of origin or to spread throughout the body. And, the surveillance system's ability to defend against cancer cells varies from patient to patient.

In other words, the term *breast cancer* does not accurately or completely describe each and every cancer of the breast. The course of the disease may be completely different in two women, even if they have the same kind of tumor. Each patient's situation must be individually evaluated and all these various factors must be considered for the disease to be accurately described.

TWO

Who Develops
Breast Cancer?

No one knows the specific cause or causes of breast cancer right now. It seems to be a disease or group of diseases found in women where a complex interrelationship of factors is present. Heredity, the effects of environment, stress, and other as-yet-unknown factors all contribute to the formation of cancerous cells.

No one can predict who will develop this disease. Thus, when we discuss those women who seem most likely to develop breast cancer, we are saying that over the course of years, physicians have learned that certain women have a higher statistical risk than others. These women should be especially watchful for the signs and symptoms of breast cancer in its earliest stages.

Certain Myths

Before discussing the risk factors involved in breast cancer, let's clear up certain myths and misconceptions which have lingered on for years. None of the following are considered to be causes of breast cancer:

- Sexual relations, fondling, caressing, or manipulation of any kind.
- Bruises, bites, bumps, or trauma to the breast.
- Having or nursing a baby. In fact, nursing a baby may make you less susceptible to developing breast cancer.
- Wearing tight brassieres or other clothing; wearing no brassiere.

In addition, breast cancer is not contagious. And large-breasted women are not more prone to developing it than other women.

Risk Factors

There are various risk factors that *are* important in considering which women may develop breast cancer:

Your Age

As with many other diseases, the longer you live, the more likely you are to develop breast cancer. The incidence of breast cancer increases as a woman enters her forties. It levels off between the ages of 45 and 55 and then rises again at a more gradual rate than it did earlier. Postmenopausal women are at the highest risk. It is important to know that eight out of ten breast cancers occur in women over the age of 45, but nowadays, physicians are seeing more and more women in their midthirties with the disease. Hopefully, this is due to earlier recognition of the problem by women and their physicians.

Previous Breast Cancer

Breast cancer may be found in both breasts, either at the same time or at different times in a woman's life. Therefore, if you have had one breast cancer, you are at risk of developing another, either in the same breast or in the other one. Various studies have shown that a significant number of women with breast cancer in one breast also develop it in the other breast. Some physicians believe that in general, if a woman has had a malignancy in one breast, her statistical chances of developing cancer in the other is increased by about 1 percent every year after that, with an overall risk increase of 5 times that of the general population.

The risk of developing another cancerous lesion depends on many factors. If the tumor is multifocal (if it tends to form in microscopic areas throughout both breasts), there is an increased chance of another tumor eventually forming. A woman with a history of breast cancer in her family (along with having her own breast cancer) may have a three-fold increase in the risk of developing cancer in the other breast.

Some physicians and researchers feel that certain types of fibrocystic disease increase a woman's chances of developing breast cancer and therefore put her at high risk. They have delineated specific types of cellular changes they consider to be *premalignant* changes, though these changes are still benign at the time of diagnosis.

The risk associated with premalignant changes is between 2½ to 5 times over the risk within the general population. It also seems that if these premalignant changes are present early in the premenopausal stage of a woman's life, they are of greater significance than such changes in an older woman's breasts.

Your Family History

Hardly anyone doubts that heredity contributes to the development of breast cancer. A woman whose mother or sister has had breast cancer is twice as prone to developing it, and there is growing evidence that a woman whose father's sister or maternal or paternal grandmother had the disease is also at high risk.

There are some modifying factors to all this. Your risk may not be much higher than average if the following facts are present:

- The breast cancer occurred in only one generation.
- The cancer was confined to one breast.
- The cancer appeared after menopause.

Suppose both your sisters had cancer but they each had it confined to only one breast and it occurred in each case before menopause. Statistically, your risk would then be about 18 percent (as compared to the normal of about 8 or 9 percent). However, if both your sisters had bilateral cancer (located in both breasts), the odds of your developing breast cancer would increase to about 50 percent.

Your genetic predisposition to breast cancer increases when the disease is diagnosed in two generations. If, for example, your mother and your grandmother each had bilateral cancer before menopause, your risk rises to about 50 percent. Again, your risk is increased only slightly if a relative had breast cancer in only one breast and if the disease developed after menopause.

A strong family history of cancer in certain organs other than the breast is also associated with an increased risk of developing breast cancer. But a family history of breast cancer is the most important kind of disease in placing you in the high-risk category.

A word of caution: Even if your family history indicates you are in a high-risk category, this does *not* mean you will develop breast cancer! We are dealing with statistics which indicate *risk,* not the disease.

Your Childbearing and Menstrual History

If you had your first child before the age of 18, you run about one-third the risk of a woman whose first child was born after she turned 35. Becoming pregnant before the age of 30 seems to offer some "protection." Women who have their first child after age 30 are at slightly higher risk than those who have *never* given birth.

Another risk factor seems to be your age at the onset of menstruation and at menopause. If you began menstruating after age 15 and reach an early menopause, your risk is reduced. On the other hand, women with a long menstrual history (early onset of menstruation and a late menopause) are at higher than average risk. In summary, the shorter your menstrual history and the more children you've had at an earlier age, the more protected you seem to be against developing breast cancer.

Female Hormones

To some extent, the development of breast cancer is related to ovarian influences and to the circulating levels of the female hormone estrogen. Hormone activity is also thought to have some relationship to the development of benign fibrocystic disease. This may answer the question about why some women with a long history of benign fibrocystic breast disease may be at higher risk of eventually developing breast cancer.

Various studies of the long-term effects of diethylstilbestrol (DES), a synthetic estrogen, and its relationship to breast cancer, have not been conclusive. In the 1940s and 1950s about 2 million women took DES to avert possible miscarriages. Any difference noted in the incidence of breast cancer in these women or in their daughters compared to women never exposed to DES has been statistically insignificant.

A government task force stated that "a relationship between DES exposure during pregnancy and the risk of cancer is unproved. However, existing studies are sufficient cause for serious concern over the drug's carcinogenic potential in this population."*

This task force recommended that research continue on the long-term effects of DES. Among other recommendations, the task force advised physicians to inform patients and their daughters who were exposed to DES of the need for long-term follow-up. It also recommended that these women examine their breasts monthly, follow the National Cancer Institute guidelines for mammography, and avoid exposure to other estrogens if possible. This includes oral contraceptives, estrogens in a "morning-after" pill, and estrogens used for replacement during or after menopause.

Although the Pill is suspected as possibly having some role in the development of breast cancer, this has not yet been determined. As a matter of fact, recent evidence indicates that women, while taking oral contraceptives, have a *lower* incidence of breast cancer than women of comparable age who do not take the Pill. The long-term effects of the Pill have not yet been completely assessed.

We are nowhere near hearing the last word on this important topic but right now, the Food and Drug Administration requires the manufacturers of oral contraceptives to include information in package inserts warning consumers of the suspected link of these medications to breast cancer.

Your Diet

Women in America and Northern Europe have five times the incidence of breast cancer as do women in Asia and Africa. The most extensive study has been among Japanese

* "DES Task Force Summary Report," National Cancer Institute, October 1978.

women. Their low incidence of breast cancer may be partly because their diets are low in animal fat and calories. When Japanese women move to Hawaii and begin eating more Western fare, their incidence of breast cancer falls somewhere between that of their homeland and those of Caucasian Americans. Moreover, when Japanese women move to mainland America and become even more Westernized in their dietary habits, the incidence of breast cancer rises dramatically and matches that of Caucasian American women.

Added to this is the fact that breast cancer occurs with much greater frequency as we go higher up the socioeconomic ladder. This correlates with affluent people consuming food richer in cholesterol and protein than do less-well-off people. Also, lower income families tend to have more children at an earlier age. This may add another factor to the complicated mosaic. At present, no one knows if the decisive factor is a general low-calorie diet or certain low-fat foods that may keep the incidence of breast cancer down. However, it does appear that diet may have something to do with the development of breast cancer.

Exposure to Radiation

High-energy radiation to the chest is associated with an increase in breast cancer. When the breasts of girls in their teens or of young women in their twenties and thirties are exposed to repeated small doses of such radiation, there is a striking increase in the number of cases of breast cancers. This was observed years ago when the treatment of tuberculosis involved frequent x-ray and fluoroscopic examinations to the affected side of the chest. Later in life, these women developed a high incidence of cancers of the breast on the irradiated side. The same evidence appears when follow-up studies were made of the long-term effects of the atomic bomb blast at Hiroshima. Japanese women exposed to this thermonuclear radiation later developed much more breast cancer as compared to other women of comparable age and cultural backgrounds.

Ethnic Origin

There is a slightly higher incidence of breast cancer among white women, American women, and Jewish women than among other women throughout the world.

It is not known how greatly any of the risk factors we have discussed contributes to an individual woman's developing breast cancer, nor is it known how they may operate in combination with each other.

You must remember that these risk factors are statistics for large groups of women. When applied to any one individual, they are less valid indicators of risk. Since the list is a long one, any woman will fit into at least one or more of these high-risk categories. This can be very misleading. Again, being in a high-risk group is *not* a sign of disease. It is a statistical indication of possible risk for a group of women over the course of their lifetimes.

While falling into any or even all of these high risks groups does not mean you will develop breast cancer, fitting into none of them does not guarantee you immunity. There is no sure way right now to tell *who* will develop the disease. Every woman, no matter which categories she does or does not fit into, is a potential victim.

❧ Barbara Conti was a 57-year-old, married grade school teacher, who discovered a breast lump 12 years earlier.* It turned out to be malignant. Let's examine her risk factors to assess her risk profile for developing breast cancer.

* All patients' names have been changed to ensure confidentiality.

She was 45 years old at the time; certainly within the age group for this disease, but not really in the *older* group. And she was *not* postmenopausal.

Barbara had no history of previous breast cancer. Nor did she have a history of benign fibrocystic disease of the breast. There was no history of breast cancer in Barbara's immediate family. A second cousin of Barbara's had developed breast cancer some years earlier, but that was the only family connection to this disease.

Barbara's childbearing and menstrual history were more in accord with the high-risk factors than any other single indicator. She had her first period at the age of 11, and at 45 was still having a regular flow. In other words, she had a "long" menstrual history. Her childbearing history was also in accord with what is termed "high risk." Barbara and her husband had long ago decided they did not wish to have children.

Barbara's dietary habits did not unduly predispose her to developing breast cancer. An attractive and trim woman, she never had weight problems. She enjoyed a diet high in protein, but that is not out of step with the diet of most Americans.

Barbara had used birth control pills for a few years and then switched to using a diaphragm.

She had never been exposed to undue amounts of radiation either as a child or an adult.

Her ethnic origin was Irish and Italian, a mixture of Northern European (a higher incidence of breast cancer) and Mediterranean stock (a somewhat lower incidence).

All in all, Barbara Conti's picture is a blend of high-, middle-, and low-risk factors. In this respect she may be "typical," since she shows that there is no real "typical" breast cancer patient.

Yet on a Monday morning 12 years ago, while showering before leaving for work, Barbara discovered a lump in her left breast. It was a hard, discrete, nonmovable, nontender mass. Barbara made an appointment that very day to see her gynecologist. We will follow Barbara and other patients throughout the rest of the book and we will see exactly what happened to her and other women with breast cancer.

Dealing with Your Risk Factors

Suppose you fit into some of the high-risk categories. How can this information help you deal with your risk of developing breast cancer?

For starters, you should learn about breast self-examination (BSE), and you should examine your breasts regularly each month (see Chapter 3). The greatest protection you can have at present is knowledge about breast cancer and the willingness to self-examine each *month*. Early detection is still the most important key to reducing the possibility of life-threatening breast cancer!

If you are within the major high-risk categories, there are other steps you may wish to take. They include the following:

* You should learn about other breast-cancer detection methods. We will detail these in the next chapter.
* If you have a strong family history of breast cancer, you may wish to avoid using oral contraceptives, although this is somewhat controversial.
* You should regularly visit your physician (at least once each year) and have a complete physical exam, including a thorough breast examination. But this is *not* a substitute for self-examination of your breasts!
* It would be wise to avoid unnecessary x-rays, especially

of the chest. This is especially important for adolescent girls, whose developing breast tissue may be affected by radiation.

- You should avoid a high-fat and high-cholesterol diet, keeping calories down and your weight to a reasonable level for your height and body build. Statistics indicate that overweight women may have a higher-than-average occurrence of breast cancer. Also, a breast lump is more difficult to detect in large, fatty breasts.
- If you are postmenopausal, you might consider minimizing the use of replacement estrogens. Although these have not been implicated in the development of breast cancer, some physicians feel it is unwise to add any more possible "risks" to an already loaded equation.

Not all the risk factors we have enumerated are given the same weight in assessing risk. Most physicians agree that the three most important are those we discussed first:

- Advanced age
- A previous breast cancer
- A family history of breast cancer

If you fall into these risk categories, you should take more precautions and be examined more often than most women in the population at large.

Frequently Asked Questions

I'm a 30-year-old woman. I had a breast augmentation last year. The doctor used silicone. Does all this put me into a high-risk category?

No, it does not. The silicone used in breast implants is a semisolid variety. There is no evidence we know of which indicates that women who have had silicone implants in their breasts have an increased incidence of breast cancer over the general population.

I have inverted nipples. Does this mean I have a greater risk of getting breast cancer?

No. Inverted nipples are fairly common. So are other differences in nipples: varying size, pigment hues, shapes, positions, and so on. None of these normal variations makes you more or less prone to developing breast cancer. However, if your nipples have recently inverted over a short period of time, it would be wise to contact your physician for a checkup.

Can men develop breast cancer?

Yes, but this is extremely rare. Men have much less breast tissue (milk glands and ducts) than women. Also, there are not the fluctuating levels of female hormones circulating in a man's system as in a woman's system during her menstrual cycle.

I've heard that cancer of the uterus is linked to breast cancer. Is this true?

Women who have had cancer of the ovary, colon, and some kinds of endometrial cancer (cancer of the uterine lining) have a greater incidence of breast cancer than the general population.

In general, a history of cancer elsewhere in the body, or a family history of cancer of organs other than the breast, may indicate a weakened immune system. While not precisely associated with breast cancer, this may be meaningful in assessing your own risk.

My mother had breast cancer at the age of 58. Am I at high risk?

In answering your question we must take into consideration *all* the important factors. It seems appropriate to consider yourself at "higher risk" than another woman whose relatives have never had breast cancer, but this is not the entire answer.

First, your mother's breast cancer occurred after her menopause, which is better than if it developed earlier. Second, if her breast cancer was in one breast only, it is better than bilateral breast cancer. We would need to know if there is any other history of breast cancer in your family, either on your mother's or your father's side. With no breast cancer in another generation on either side of the family, your statistical risk is lower than if there is such a history. Although you may be at some increased risk, you should not overestimate that risk. Remember, statistics do not tell the entire story.

I'm 30 years old. I hear that more and more younger women are getting breast cancer. Is this true?

It is statistically true that more young women are having the diagnosis of breast cancer made than ever before. This does not necessarily mean that breast cancer is on the rise. It may simply reflect more general awareness of the disease, more women self-examining at younger ages and finding lumps, and better detection and screening methods. You should react to this kind of information by keeping in mind that you are an individual with a specific family, genetic, and life history. Statistics reflect general population trends and can be misleading when applied to any one person.

Does stress cause or influence breast cancer?

This is a difficult question to answer with any certainty. Psychiatrists and other physicians have long known that stress, anxiety, depression, and major emotional disruptions in peoples' lives are often associated with many different illnesses.

Prolonged emotional stress may lead to or aggravate medical conditions as diverse as ulcers, arthritis, asthma, allergies, disorders of the colon, hypertension, heart disease, and many others. It is not possible to directly link up emotional stress to cancer, but most physicians agree that prolonged emotional turmoil can be debilitating and may alter various immune mechanisms. This may, in turn, make people more susceptible to illnesses varying in severity from cancer to the common cold.

I've heard that a virus can cause breast cancer. Is this true?

It is well recognized that in certain strains of mice, breast cancer can be transmitted from mothers to daughters. If the female offspring of these mice are separated from their mothers and fed artificially or by foster parents, they do not develop the disease. The milk of these maternal mice has been shown to contain a virus known as the Bitner virus, which is clearly associated with breast cancer in these *mice.* However, there is no substantive evidence from human studies that breast cancer is transmitted by this route. There is no need to worry that viral infections such as encountered in a common cold or sore throat may lead to breast cancer.

I'm 32 years old and childless. I had an abortion nine years ago. Does this make me less prone to getting breast cancer than a woman who has never been pregnant?

It is generally accepted that having a child while you are young reduces your risk of developing breast cancer. This "protection" is seen only in women who have had a *full-term* pregnancy resulting in the delivery of a child. Statistically, there is a slightly greater incidence of breast cancer in women who have had abortions than in those who have not. These statistics seem to hold true for older women, even those past the age of 75.

I'm 50 years old and am taking estrogens as replacement therapy. Does this increase my chance of developing breast cancer?

This question has not been answered completely or to our satisfaction. Many studies to date have failed to show any correlation between estrogen replacement therapy and breast cancer. Some studies have suggested that there is a slightly increased risk among women who have taken estrogens for menopausal and postmenopausal symptoms for a period of time greater than 10 years. Among these women, the incidence was highest for those who used very high-dose tablets and who developed benign fibrocystic breast disease after beginning hormone replacement therapy.

Most physicians would probably agree that if you fall into the major high-risk categories, you should not use estrogens for replacement therapy. Furthermore, it is generally advised by conservative physicians that if estrogen replacement therapy is used, it should not be administered in high doses for a prolonged period of time since there is a *possibility* of an increase in the risk of breast cancer.

I smoke two packs of cigarettes a day. Does this increase my chances of getting breast cancer?

Although cigarette smoking has been linked with lung, bladder, cervical, and stomach cancer, as well as with a variety of other serious diseases, we know of no studies to date linking cigarettes with an increased incidence of breast cancer.

I exercise regularly using Nautilus equipment. Will building up my chest muscles possibly increase my chances of developing breast cancer?

No. When exercised, chest muscles, which lie beneath the breast tissue, may increase in size and thereby make your breasts appear more prominent, but we know of no danger to your breasts because of such exercises.

THREE

Detecting
a Lump

Until breast cancer can be prevented, the greatest hope for its control is early detection of a suspicious lesion. This must then be followed, of course, by accurate diagnosis and treatment. In this chapter we will discuss breast lumps, their detection, what they may (and may not) mean, and the most important tools you have at your disposal for detecting anything abnormal about your breasts.

To begin with, about 80 percent of all breast lumps are completely benign. As we've already said, the most common cause of breast lumps in women between the ages of 35 and 55 is benign fibrocystic disease. Unlike most cancer lumps, these are usually smooth in contour, easily movable within the breast, and are often fairly soft. They may give the breast a nodular feeling. They are often multiple and may occur in both breasts.

🌷 Ann Snyder was a 39-year-old woman whose mother had been treated for breast cancer 8 years earlier. Although her mother had done very well, Ann lived in a state of constant worry about the possibility that she herself might develop the disease. She had visited several physicians, asking them to examine her breasts for any suspicious lumps or masses. None were found. On the surface, Ann seemed to be a woman who would not hesitate to carefully examine her breasts and who would take immediate action if she found anything suspicious.

While showering one evening, she discovered a small spherical, movable lump in her left breast. Horrified, she became acutely anxious. She called a friend and discussed the situation with her. Over the next 3 months, fearful she now had cancer, Ann made several appointments with her physician, but backed down each time. Finally, with her friend and husband becoming increasingly concerned about Ann's escalating anxiety, she did go to her doctor.

Ann's lump was aspirated. The diagnosis was definite: She had a benign cyst. Because of her anxiety and fear of a diagnosis of cancer, Ann had spent needless months in terror. After the aspiration biopsy, Ann made plans for regular follow-up and learned about breast self-examination.

Ann's story is not unusual. Many women fear they may "find something" and spend needless months, or longer, enduring a host of frightening fantasies about breast cancer. We will have more to say about this later in this chapter. There are a number of benign breast conditions that may make you think you have cancer. The only sure-fire method of knowing the exact diagnosis is by microscopic evaluation of the tissue.

It is helpful to know the signs and symptoms that may indicate breast cancer. The most important thing to remember is that after you are 20 years old, any lump in the breast should be thoroughly investigated. Here are the things to watch for:

- A lump. A single, painless lump in the breast is the most common sign of cancer. Before you are 30 years old, the most likely cause of a lump is a benign, fibrocystic mass. After menopause, the appearance of a lump may indeed mean cancer.
- Inversion of the nipple. This may mean cancer unless, of course, the nipple in question was always inverted. A tumor located beneath the nipple may be difficult to feel, and it may be the nipple retraction rather than a lump that you will first notice. Such a retraction can be seen much more easily when your arms are raised.
- Puckering or dimpling of the breast. A tumor does not always form a round lump. Instead, it may form an area of thickening so that the tissue leading from deep in the breast to the skin becomes involved. This may pull on the skin and form a pucker or dimple. This can be best seen by looking in the mirror and raising your arms above your head. Or it may become more evident if you place your hands on your hips and apply pressure to the hips, which tightens the chest muscles.
- Swelling of the breast. Some tumors cause the entire breast to swell. The breast may be heavy and swollen, and the skin appears swollen. When this occurs, the skin pores become more easily visible and make the skin look like that of an orange. This "orange skin" is very characteristic of skin in which fluid is retained and where inflammation is present.
- Swelling or a lump in the armpit. Even if there is no obvious abnormality in your breast, a lump in the armpit may be a sign of cancer. This may mean there is a small,

deeply situated tumor within your breast. It may be too deep within the tissue to be felt, but it has spread to the axillary lymph nodes on that side of the body. You should visit your physician immediately.

- Pain in the breast. Breast cancer is usually painless, but pain frequently brings women to their physicians. The most frequent cause of breast pain is benign fibrocystic breast disease. Here, the pain and tenderness are cyclic, increasing in the premenstrual phase of your cycle. It is usually bilateral, although often more pronounced on one side, and is most marked in the upper, outer portions of the breasts. Many women describe such pain by saying, "My breasts feel heavy and tender, as if they're filled with milk." However, there *are* some cases of breast cancer where the first symptom is breast pain, so if you experience pain or breast discomfort that you never before had, a visit to your doctor is in order.
- Nipple discharge. There are many kinds of discharges. The most serious is a bloody discharge or one where blood and watery fluid are mixed together, usually coming from one breast. Certain benign breast tumors may cause a bloody discharge from one breast. A discharge together with a palpable lump may be an important combination of signs indicating cancer. Such a discharge should be examined microscopically by a pathologist, and a thorough search for any cancer cells should be made.
- Nipple irritation or elevation of the nipple. A persistent scaly or eczemalike irritation of the skin of the nipple may be a sign of Paget's disease, a form of cancer affecting the milk ducts and overlying skin. Elevation of the nipple may be due to a benign tumor but it may also indicate breast cancer.

- In general, any change in the consistency or size or shape of the breast and any change in the color, texture, or quality of the breast skin, of the nipple, or of the areola should be promptly reported to your physician.

It is important to emphasize again that about 80 percent of breast tumors are benign! Many of the signs and symptoms we have described may indicate benign tumors or cysts that are of no consequence. Or they may be the first important changes indicating breast cancer. It is not possible for you to tell the difference by wondering about it or by constantly reexamining such findings on your own. To be certain about what you have, you must visit your physician! Only the appropriate examination and tests will give you the answer. You should act promptly to eliminate guesswork and worrisome speculation from your thinking.

Breast Self-Examination: A Crucial Issue

In our opinion, breast self-examination (BSE) is the most important issue when dealing with breast cancer. Here are the reasons why:

The highest cure rates are obtained if a breast tumor is discovered when it is pea-sized or smaller. This is the minimum size at which a mass can be felt by you or your doctor on physical examination. On the other hand, the survival rate from breast cancer drops to about 45 percent if the tumor is discovered later, when it is 1 to 2 inches wide, and when the axillary lymph nodes have become involved.

Again and again, studies show that early detection by self-examination (either coupled with screening procedures such as mammography or alone) results in more successful treatment. Smaller cancers with less involvement of lymph nodes, picked up in women who have consistently done self-examination, results in a very significant reduction of deaths from breast cancer. These findings are confirmed by 5-, 7-, and 10-year follow-up studies.

Self-examination is crucial because over 90 percent of breast cancer signs are discovered by women themselves, either by accident or through regular examination. Included in this 90 percent figure are tumors discovered by husbands or partners. You cannot depend on once- or twice-a-year visits to your doctor. You must regularly self-examine each month!

Unfortunately, too few women practice this vital routine. A Gallup study commissioned by the American Cancer Society revealed that more than three-quarters of the women surveyed were aware of breast self-examination but only 18 percent practiced it on a regular monthly basis. A follow-up study 3 years later showed only a slight increase in this figure. What can we learn from this important statistic?

For one thing, we think that *how* a woman learns about BSE affects how frequently she practices it. The Gallup study indicated that one-third of the women who were aware of BSE had received personal instruction by a physician, nurse, or other health professional. Among those who received personal instruction, 92 percent practiced BSE, and 33 percent said they practiced it regularly each month.

How can we account for the fact that so many women, although knowing about BSE, do not practice it and may not go to their physicians even after discovering a breast lump?

A recent study in Great Britain showed that the over-whelming majority of women with lumps in their breasts had intentionally delayed reporting their symptoms to a family doctor. The delay varied from a few months to several years. In most cases ignorance was not responsible for the delay. Rather, most women admitted it was *fear* of having the diagnosis of cancer made. They simply wanted to delay or not look at what they thought would be the inevitable bad news. And this overwhelming fear persisted even though only 20 percent of breast tumors turn out to be cancer. Far too many women live in dread of cancer and the "inevitable" when all they really have is a benign breast mass, which can be diagnosed quickly by a physician.

It is the responsibility of every physician to educate women about BSE. If your physician does not initiate or encourage you to learn BSE, you should request it. Do not hesitate!

Let's return to the reasons why so many women avoid breast self-examination. The Gallup study showed certain other important statistics that lead us to believe that women may neglect themselves for a number of reasons.

- A lack of complete knowledge. Many women in the study were simply not aware that BSE should be done *monthly*. More than one-third of the women who knew about BSE but did not practice it mistakenly believed that a yearly examination by a physician is sufficient. More than half the women surveyed did not know that any specific position(s) should be assumed during BSE, and one-third did not know what possible signs of breast cancer to watch out for.

- A lack of confidence. Despite having learned to do BSE, only one in five women who practiced it felt certain about what they were doing. Only one-third felt sure they would know what a lump would feel like. Lack of confidence and a sense of uncertainty are not unusual when people are treading on unfamiliar ground, but confidence in your ability to do BSE can be gained through regular and thorough practice.

- Fear and anxiety. As we've already mentioned, fear about what may be found makes some women ignore themselves and not perform BSE. Nearly half the women surveyed felt that a monthly examination would make them worry unnecessarily. Others simply said, "I just don't have the time," or "I don't really need it." Psychiatrists call this kind of response *denial*. Many people use denial to protect themselves from unpleasant thoughts or feelings. In a sense, they say, "I'm not going to look at this; therefore, it's not really there." It means closing your eyes to reality and is the least adaptive way you can face a real or potentially real problem in your life. Many women are fearful that the diagnosis of cancer guarantees disfigurement. They fail to recognize that with earlier detection it is possible to have less extensive surgery as part of the treatment. And today, with new reconstruction techniques, breast cancer surgery need not result in life-long deformity or mutilation.

- Various psychological taboos. Some women may be reluctant to practice BSE thoroughly because they are embarrassed about it. They may liken it to something they mistakenly feel is sinful, such as masturbation, or a sign of inappropriate narcissism. Others may think it's a sign of hypochondria, that to self-examine means being overly concerned or worried about one's health. Some may simply think it's wrong to touch their own breasts. More public education is needed to teach women about BSE and also to reinforce its social acceptability.

- Fatalism. We have all seen fatalism in our daily lives. "If I'm going to get it, that's that and nothing will help me. So why bother about it?" Such fatalistic thinking ignores the fact that self-examination may detect breast cancer before it has metastasized and when it can be treated most effectively.

These reasons why women ignore BSE and the possibility of breast cancer, along with our own experiences with patients, have prompted us to reorient our thinking as follows:

Some time ago it was assumed that because many women came to physicians with large breast lumps, medical science was dealing with an invariably fatal and rapidly progressing disease. We no longer believe this.

We believe these figures indicate a failure of the medical community and of the general public to recognize the crucial role of early detection of breast cancer. Until recently, this vital public health issue has not been addressed completely. In our view, ignoring what breast symptoms may (and may not) mean, pretending everything is fine, and failing to teach and to learn all we can about breast cancer represent a failure of concerned commitment on the parts of the medical community, the health delivery system, and women themselves.

Here is the crux of the situation: You must know about breast cancer and about BSE now, *before* you think you may ever develop the disease. We believe this public health issue deserves the highest possible priority. We believe the facts about breast cancer and BSE should be taught to every young woman in an organized public forum. This information and a course on BSE should be part of every high school girl's organized curriculum, just as are hygiene or gym class. Surely, breast cancer, with its impact on millions of women and their families, is no less important.

Examining Your Breasts

Examining your breasts is the most certain way of protecting yourself against breast cancer. *You* are the most important part of this equation. Before describing this examination, a few words of encouragement and caution are in order.

By examining your breasts each month you are *not* trying to be a cancer expert. You are not taking over your doctor's role. You will simply look for any breast *changes* that may or may not be significant. If you find a change, you should then seek prompt attention from a physician.

We have heard many patients say, "I don't know what I'm supposed to be looking for . . . I'm not a doctor." Or "My breasts are lumpy already . . . they always have been. How am I supposed to find a new lump?" If you lack confidence in your ability to do BSE, make certain to get a thorough breast examination from your physician. Watch the doctor's technique carefully. Do more than just watch; ask questions! Ask your doctor to show you the proper method of examination. Then, do the examination yourself with your doctor watching. Spend enough time so when you leave the office you feel you have a head start in learning BSE technique.

Don't be reluctant to ask your physician questions and to ask to be taught BSE. Any physician genuinely interested in patients will welcome such questions and will gladly instruct you in the correct technique. There is no reason to be shy or embarrassed. The medical community has now taken a very active role in educating patients in BSE. Life-size dolls and models are available to simulate breast masses so women can have a better idea about what to look for.

If you get to know your own breasts thoroughly through regular, deliberate examination, you will become more familiar with *your* own normal anatomy than any physician could ever be. Getting to know your breast contours in their normal condition will help you know what may be abnormal.

When to Examine

Examine your breasts at the same time every month. This will help you make BSE a habit. If you are premenopausal, this is very important because there will be monthly cyclic changes in the size and texture of your breasts. Your breasts will appear larger and will be more tender just before your period. Recognizing these cyclic changes will prevent your becoming frightened if you suddenly discover something which is nothing more than a normal variation in your breast tissue. Also, examining your breasts at the same time each month will give you a consistent baseline for comparison each time you self-examine.

The best time to examine yourself is several days after the end of your last period, when your breasts are probably not swollen or tender. If you are postmenopausal, when you do it is not important since there are no longer the fluctuations in hormone levels. However, if you do your examination on the same day of the month, BSE is more likely to become a routine habit.

Keeping a record of your self-examinations inside a medicine cabinet or next to any medication you take regularly will serve as a reminder.

Set aside enough time and go through the steps slowly and deliberately. It may be helpful at first to make up a checklist of the steps and, as you repeat them, actually check off the steps. The only good examination is a complete one!

The Examination

Breast self-examination is really quite simple. You should stand before a mirror with your right arm behind your head. Then with your left hand, using two or three fingers, gently explore your right breast. Use gentle but firm pressure and go in a clockwise motion, starting at the nipple and moving outward until you have palpated the entire breast. You should be feeling for any unusual lump or mass beneath the skin. You must also feel into the right armpit, trying to detect any lumps there. This should then be repeated on the other side.

Next, still standing in front of the mirror, inspect your breasts for anything unusual (size, color, skin texture, dimpling, puckering, inversion of a nipple, and so on). Firmly pressing your palms together in front of your chin will accentuate any dimpling; so will placing your hands on your hips and pressing downward. You should also inspect your breasts with your arms at your sides, with your arms raised above your head, and while bending forward at the waist. Then, press each nipple gently and look for any discharge.

The fingertip examination, or palpation, should then be repeated on both breasts while you are lying flat on your back. This flattens your breast tissue, allowing any deeper mass to be palpated. Again, when examining the right breast and armpit, your right hand should be kept behind your head as you feel with the fingertips of your left hand. The reverse is true when examining your left breast.

You may find it easier to palpate your breasts in the standing position while in the shower. Soapy fingers will glide easily over your wet skin. But you should still perform the examination in the lying-down position after your shower.

If you are large-breasted, you may have some trouble conducting a thorough examination. You may find it helpful to steady the outside of each breast by bracing it against a solid surface.

Women with small breasts may sometimes mistake a rib for a lump. If you feel something hard beneath your breast, follow the lump with your fingers to the center line of your body, feeling where the rib joins the sternum. This will let you determine if the "lump" you felt was a rib.

The entire examination in the standing and lying positions should take between 10 and 15 minutes.

A few additional words about breast lumps may help you differentiate benign fibrocystic disease from something more serious.

As described above, cancer is often, though not always, a single, hard, painless lump that does not change size or shape during the menstrual cycle. It often occurs in the upper, outer section of the breast and more often, in the left breast.

Cysts and other benign growths may be painful. They may occur in both breasts, and they may be multiple. They often vary in size and painfulness depending on the stage of your menstrual cycle. And they are often slightly movable. A cancerous lump is usually not movable, because it tends to invade surrounding tissue and become fixed since that tissue forms scars and adheres to the tumor. Cancer may be accompanied by hard, irregular nodes in the armpit or by dimpling or inversion of the nipple.

These general rules are not a complete guide as to which lump or mass is important and which is not. *Any* lump or change should be promptly investigated!

Other Methods of Detection

In the last few years researchers have developed a number of sophisticated devices for diagnosing a malignancy and for detecting hidden tumors before they become palpable. These techniques include the following:

Mammography

This process, which involves x-raying the breast, has received the most attention and has been found to be very useful in cases where a tumor has already been palpated. The technique can also detect tumors smaller than those palpable by hand, and it gives information as to the possible malignancy of a mass. Mammography has been reported to be 95 percent accurate with tumor masses that are in the 1 centimeter range.

A mammographic examination is performed by a radiologist, although the operation of the machine may be done by a trained radiologic technician. Two exposures at right angles are made of each breast. The entire breast is visible in the mammograms, which are then analyzed by a radiologist. A report is sent to the referring physician, who will probably recommend a biopsy if cancer is suspected.

Two important studies have pointed out the advantages and drawbacks of mammography as a screening device, although no one questions the value of mammography when it is used for the diagnosis of women who already have symptomatic findings.

The Health Insurance Plan of Greater New York (HIP), in cooperation with the National Cancer Institute, began a controlled clinical trial to determine if yearly screening of women with no cancer symptoms would help reduce deaths from breast cancer in women over the age of 50. Thirty-one thousand women were given a free annual screening mammography and physical examination and were compared to another group of 31,000 who received no unusual screening or care.

The results of the study were very revealing. In the group over 50 years of age, breast cancer mortality was reduced by over 40 percent; below age 40 there was no difference in mortality rates between the study and control groups. The combination of physical examination *and* yearly mammography was effective in lowering mortality rates in older, symptom-free women who were later found to have cancer.

Based on this study, the National Cancer Institute and the American Cancer Society jointly sponsored 27 Breast

Cancer Detection Demonstration Projects (BCDDPs). Their aim was to monitor a total of 280,000 women between the ages of 35 and 74 by physical examination, mammography, and thermography (photographs of the breast's heat patterns) for 5 consecutive years, with a 5-year follow-up.

During this study, concern about the possible cancer hazard posed by repeated exposure to yearly radiation led to the establishment of guidelines for breast screening by mammography. These guidelines, which are still in effect, are as follows:

- You should do monthly breast self-examination. Any abnormal findings should be reported to your physician.
- You should have an annual examination with thorough palpation of the breasts by qualified medical personnel.
- You should not have a mammography under age 35 unless you have signs and symptoms of breast cancer.
- Between ages 35 and 39 you may have annual mammography only if you yourself have a history of breast cancer.
- Between ages 40 and 49 you may have annual mammography if you have a family history of breast cancer. Some physicians feel that one mammogram is indicated at this point so it may be compared to subsequent mammograms if they are done. This is called a baseline mammogram.
- Over age 50, annual mammography may be considered.

The effects of radiation exposure from mammography are difficult to determine. The ideal maximum radiation dosage per examination per breast is less than 1 rad (absorbed dose of radiation). With new methods, good quality mammograms can now be obtained with doses of 0.2 to 0.3 rad. Even more sophisticated techniques (delivering as little as .05 rad to each breast per complete examination) are being investigated. It appears that considerably reduced radiation dosage is going to become available, and the risks involved in mammography may be much less than those a few years ago.

There is no doubt that in these studies, mammography coupled with thorough annual examination detected smaller, less advanced breast cancers with a lower incidence of lymph node involvement. However, some physicians have reservations about the results of these studies and about mammography as a screening method. These reservations are:

- There may be a higher-than-expected incidence of breast cancers in the screened population in these studies because many women may have used the screening clinics as an opportunity to come forward with a breast lump they had known about for some time. Some researchers also feel that the studies encouraged women who knew they were in the high-risk groups for breast cancer to come forward. If this *did* happen, the results of these studies may not be an accurate reflection of the population at large.
- A negative finding on any one screening examination may create in some women a false sense of security. This may unwittingly encourage them to avoid self-examination and an annual examination by a physician.
- Screening programs using mammography will often generate more breast biopsies than would otherwise occur since many women with benign breast lumps will be screened and referred to surgeons. Even the smallest breast operation is stressful to a patient and may be a source of considerable anxiety.
- Many abnormalities of marginal significance may be detected when studying any large group of women. The

microscopic diagnosis of breast cancer is not always a clear-cut situation, and often the surgeon and the pathologist have doubts. Some researchers are concerned that owing to large screening programs, more treatment will be done because abnormalities have been found that, if left alone, would probably never progress to invasive cancer.

• Some researchers and epidemiologists point out that large-scale screening programs are not cost-effective when we consider the expenses involved in the ultrasophisticated diagnostic equipment and the enormous monetary outlays made for professional salaries and other personnel. This points out something about statistics and large groups of people.

Any woman, when facing the possibility of breast cancer, is facing the disease as one individual. For her and her family, the stakes are *100 percent*. The cost-effectiveness ratios and cost-per-patient figures do not matter. But such things do matter to hospitals and governments, which find themselves strapped with enormously costly health care programs and with limited financial resources. Statistics are not individual people!

Many experts feel that the best thing to do is to accurately define those women who fall into high-risk groups rather than generally screen *every* woman between the ages of 30 and 70. In our view, public education would be an important and cost-effective method of bringing such high-risk women into physicians' offices and into clinic centers, where they can be screened for breast cancer and then helped.

As for these high-risk candidates, most experts today agree that childless women, over the age of 30, with a personal or family history of breast cancer are the most likely to benefit from regular mammography screening programs. As we said earlier, very few experts doubt the usefulness of mammography in diagnosing breast cancer in women who *already* have symptoms of the disease. Any existing controversy concerns the usefulness of mammography as a widespread screening technique for the population at large.

Ultrasound

Ultrasound is a method of detection, which projects high-frequency sound waves into the breast. Such sound waves when focused at a specific site will return an echo pattern depending on the size and density of the object they encounter. Within breast tissue, these sound waves will travel unimpeded through a fluid-filled cyst but will bounce back from a solid tumor that may be cancerous. The pattern of echoes from these sound waves is converted by computer into an image of the interior of the breast.

Ultrasound has its limitations. For one, it gives about 8 percent false-negative results (incorrect indications that no abnormality is present) and gives a great many false-positive results (an incorrect indication that an abnormality *is* present)—about 18 percent. Ultrasound cannot yet tell the difference between a solid tumor that is benign and one that is malignant. It visualizes tumors better in the breasts of younger women than it does in those of older women, because older women's breasts have more fat content.

Though ultrasound will miss a good many breast tumors, it is still being evaluated and may undergo further refinement for more use in the future. Some physicians believe it may help women with dense breasts or those with fibrocystic breast disease. Most important, there is no ionizing radiation.

Therefore, with improvements it may become very useful for pregnant women with breast lumps and for those under the age of 30 with breast problems.

Thermography

A mass can be analyzed by thermography. In this process, the heat patterns on the surface of the breast are converted into a picture. Rapidly growing tumors (those with a high level of cell division) have an increased blood supply and increased venous drainage. Therefore, the skin overlying them will often have a higher surface temperature resulting in infrared radiation from the skin. In a thermographic picture, an abnormality is represented by a "hot spot," which is an increased area of blood supply.

To have a thermogram you must undress above the waist and then wait in a room that is, at most, 68 degrees Fahrenheit until your skin temperature cools. You must hold your arms away from your body (above your head or out at the sides) for 10 minutes so that any possible "hot spots" located within the breasts or axilla are not masked by ordinary body heat. Then, your breasts are photographed by an infrared camera that records skin surface temperatures.

The advantage of thermography is that it does not involve ionizing radiation. Since mammograms are not recommended for symptom-free women under the age of 40, women with a family history of breast cancer but who have no palpable breast lump may be periodically examined by this method.

However, thermography is not really an accurate detection method at this time. It involves a highly subjective evaluation by the radiologist and may detect less than half of all tumors. Although one study indicated that women with abnormal thermograms have a fifteenfold increased risk of developing breast cancer, an abnormal thermogram alone is not considered sufficient cause for a woman to then have a biopsy. And a normal thermogram is not considered reliable enough to indicate that all is well. Refinement in the machines being used and standardization of thermogram readings have not yet been achieved. Until these improvements occur, thermography cannot be considered a dependable and objective screening device.

Computerized Tomographic Mammography

Axial tomography may soon become a widely used tool for cancer detection. The CAT scan (computerized axial tomography) involves taking a series of pictures at various depths and angles through a portion of the body. This enables the radiologist to obtain a comprehensive image of that area since the series of pictures is like slicing a loaf of bread and having each slice pictorially represent a segment of the area.

In tomographic mammography, a contrast enhancement technique is used. Iodide material is injected into the body and is preferentially taken up by breast cancer cells. This is also seen on the CAT scan x-ray.

The CAT scan mammogram is superior to regular mammography for detecting small lesions in premenopausal women, especially when there have been minor breast changes, such as benign fibrocystic breast disease. It is most helpful when a conventional mammogram and physical examination have been inconclusive. It may very well be a promising tool because of its ability to detect extremely small cancers within the breast. However, right now, the cost of this test is so great that it is not yet suitable as a general screening method for breast cancer.

*   *   *

Each of these methods of detection has its drawbacks and advantages. And each may or may not do the proper job in any individual woman's case. We treated a patient who had a small lump on the upper, inner area of her right breast. She was examined by her physician, who then referred her for a mammogram. The test was negative. The surgeon, still suspicious, biopsied the tumor. It was a malignant cancer. All of this simply shows that no detection method is absolutely foolproof.

Frequently Asked Questions

I'm 35 years old and I'm pregnant for the first time. How do I continue to examine my breasts each month? And what about after my baby is born? I plan to breast-feed.

As more and more women over the age of 35 are choosing to have babies, many for the first time, this question is important.

During pregnancy your breasts are preparing for their function of providing your infant with milk. They enlarge progressively as the pregnancy proceeds. As a result, it is more difficult to properly examine them as you near term. You will be facing some of the difficulty a large-breasted woman may face when doing BSE. You may find it helpful to rest the outer surface of the breast against a solid surface. The technique of BSE is the same as when you were not pregnant. You must proceed deliberately through the inspection and palpation phases of the examination looking for any changes from the preceding examination.

While you are nursing your child, you will have to keep the same considerations in mind, since your breasts will be larger and fuller than ordinarily. There is no reason for you to discontinue doing BSE during this period of time.

I've heard of the Breast Pap test. What exactly is it?

The Breast Pap test is used by some physicians to detect the earliest possible signs of breast cancer. It is similar to the Pap test used to determine the earliest stages of cervical cancer. In this test, breast fluid is analyzed for abnormal cells. If the breasts are gently massaged or if a suction device is placed to the nipple, fluid may be extracted. Most body fluids will contain a few cells that have sloughed off during the natural course of events. The cells in this fluid may then be examined microscopically for evidence of cancer cells. Cancer cells, if present, will appear "atypical"; that is, the nucleus of the cell will appear misshapen and many cells will appear to be in the process of dividing.

This method has the advantage of being simple and relatively inexpensive, but since many women do not produce any fluid under the circumstances described, very few cancers are diagnosed by the Breast Pap test.

I've always had very lumpy breasts. I have trouble examining them because I'm not sure what I should be looking for. Another lump would feel the same, wouldn't it?

Many women have lumpy or nodular breasts. This is a normal variation but can make you somewhat unsure about what you are to detect when you self-examine.

Remember, you are looking for change. As we have stated, by becoming familiar with the size, shape, and feel of your own breasts through regular BSE, you will quickly recognize any change that may occur.

Though your breasts are lumpy, the chances are that if a cancerous lump appears, it will not be of the same consistency as the other nodules of normal breast tissue. As we have discussed, cancer is often a discrete, hard, nonpainful lump that does not move and that is distinctly different than normal nodules within the breast.

In an extreme case where your breasts may be so nodular that it is difficult to tell when a change occurs, your physician may suggest that you consider a subcutaneous mastectomy with immediate reconstruction. You might consider this procedure if your breast nodularity causes you enormous concern and if you have a very strong family history of breast cancer. We will talk more about this treatment in Chapter 6.

What is the risk of having any long-term effects from radiation due to mammography?

No one can accurately answer this question at this time. There are, however, many indicators that the risks, if any, are minimal and becoming less with each passing year. The possible risks are lowest to women over 30 years of age and are long-term, say 20 years, so if you are in the older age categories, there is less to worry about.

Keep in mind that more sophisticated equipment is being developed each year and that today's radiation dosage is lower than that of even a year or two ago.

At the time of this writing, the same guidelines for mammography are still in effect. However, a number of physicians, recognizing the very low radiation emitted by the newest machines, think that yearly mammography will soon be a standard procedure for *any* woman over 40 years of age, perhaps within the next year or two.

· FOUR ·

I've Found a Lump—
What Do I Do?

If you discover a breast lump or notice some other change in your breast, you must take the appropriate steps. The first step obviously involves visiting a physician. But which physician should you see?

If your relationship with your family doctor is a good one, you may want to begin there. Or you may prefer to go to your gynecologist, since he or she deals with breast lumps quite frequently. Indeed, many gynecologists are very proficient at examining breasts and will refer their patients for further diagnostic investigation when it is necessary.

Whichever physician you initially visit, you will probably be referred to someone who deals with breast lumps every day. This will most likely be a surgeon. You should clearly tell the referring physician that you wish to be sent to a surgeon who is open-minded about treatment and who will explain *all* treatment options to you if treatment becomes necessary.

There is no need for panic or alarm. You are just having a diagnosis made. In fact, the diagnostic tests done by the surgeon may be the only treatment you may need. And remember that the vast majority of breast lumps are completely benign.

Although the surgeon's only goal at this point is quick and accurate diagnosis, don't be surprised if he or she brings up the possibility that the tumor *may* be malignant. If the surgeon takes a team approach to the treatment of breast cancer, he or she may mention the name of a radiotherapist or an oncologist (a physician who specializes in the medical treatment of various cancers) to ensure a thorough evaluation of the tumor and to provide a comprehensive treatment plan if it is necessary. Surgeons are well aware of the emotionally charged nature of breast cancer, and most surgeons probably expect that their patients will *already* have some strong feelings and ideas about treatment even before any diagnosis is made. However, it is up to you at this point to make your surgeon aware of your interest in knowing all the details of your diagnosis and of your wish to have *all* possible treatment options thoroughly explained to you. (We will have more to say about these options and about a team approach to treating breast cancer in Chapter 6).

Your input is very important in helping the doctor make an accurate diagnosis. You will be asked certain questions. Is the lump painful? How long have you noticed it? How quickly or slowly has it grown? Does it vary in size, painfulness, or texture from one time of the month to another? The more you are aware of your own body and its changes, the better able you are to help your physician arrive at a diagnosis.

The doctor will carefully examine your breasts. This may include transilluminating your breast, pressing a flashlightlike instrument against the breast to try to determine if the lump is a cyst or a solid material. A benign, fluid-filled cyst will appear clear or semiclear, while a tumor appears opaque. If there is a nipple discharge, your doctor may arrange for a cytologic examination, or examination of the fluid for abnormal cells. Although this examination is not a totally foolproof means of assessing a lump, it may help indicate what the next diagnostic test should be.

Your physician may arrange for you to have a mammogram. If you have a palpable lump in your breast or under your arm (in the axilla) or have noticed any change or abnormality in the breast skin or nipple, a mammogram can help determine what the next step should be. This procedure also evaluates the tissue of the opposite breast for any changes.

Biopsy

A biopsy is the only accurate way to diagnose a suspicious lump. It is the definitive step in determining what (if anything) is to be done next. There are two kinds of biopsies, a needle biopsy and a surgical biopsy.

Needle Biopsy

A needle biopsy will help determine if a breast mass is a cyst or a tumor. It is most often done on an outpatient basis and does not require general anesthesia. Usually a surgeon does the biopsy.

There are two types of needle biopsies: a fine needle biopsy and a wide needle biopsy. In a fine needle biopsy, a syringe is used to remove fluid from the tumor. Anesthetic is not usually required. Samples of the tissue fluid are spread on a glass slide and examined microscopically by a pathologist. This examination will reveal if any cancerous cells are present. If the growth is a noncancerous cyst, it may be drained during this diagnostic process. Some surgeons may choose to simply observe the cyst at that time, not aspirating (draining) it, but rather, waiting to see what may happen. Sometimes these cysts resolve and disappear by themselves. If the cystic fluid contains cancerous cells, further treatment is in order.

A wide needle biopsy removes a small piece of tissue from the breast mass. It usually requires a local anesthetic and may be done in the office. There is one major drawback to this method: The extracted tissue specimen may not contain any evidence of cancer. However, this does not totally exclude the diagnosis of breast cancer. A cancerous section of the tumor may have been missed by the needle. In such circumstances, if it is suspected that the tumor is cancerous, the surgeon may suggest a surgical biopsy.

Surgical Biopsy

Surgical removal of a suspicious lump for evaluation (an excisional biopsy) is the primary diagnostic technique by which a definite diagnosis of cancer can be made. It can be performed under local anesthesia in a surgeon's office or may be done under general anesthesia in the hospital or on an outpatient basis. The kind of anesthesia used depends on the size and location of the mass.

There are two ways in which the excised tissue may be examined. The quicker way is by frozen section, while the patient is still anesthetized. The other method is called a permanent section. This involves a 48-hour-long process in which the tissue is fixed in formalin, imbedded in paraffin blocks, then sliced into extremely thin sections, stained, and placed under a microscope where it is studied for evidence of cancer.

Studying and diagnosing the tumor by a frozen section

allows the biopsy and any surgery that may be needed to be combined in one procedure. On the other hand, a permanent section allows for a more detailed and definitive analysis of the tissue and gives the patient and her surgeon more time and opportunity to discuss her situation and the various treatment methods available.

Over the last few years a number of important changes have occurred in performing surgical biopsies. For years, the rule of thumb had been that all biopsies were done in the operating room with the patient totally asleep. A frozen section was done, and if the tumor proved to be cancerous, a mastectomy was done right then and there. Often, with this process, a woman underwent anesthesia for a biopsy with no idea of what the results would be. She could then awake to the fact that she did have cancer and had already had a mastectomy.

This procedure is rarely done today. Most physicians do only a permanent section first. A definitive treatment, if needed, is done at a later time. In most instances where a lump is investigated, no further treatment is needed. The lump turns out to be a benign cyst. The biopsy itself (whether done by needle or by incision) cures the problem.

If the biopsy reveals that the lump under investigation is a cancerous tumor, the interval between the biopsy and treatment allows you time to make the necessary practical and emotional adjustments to the idea of cancer. You can arrange for time off from work for your treatment and recuperation. If a mastectomy is going to be done, you may wish to consult with a plastic surgeon about breast reconstruction, which can be performed soon after the mastectomy or even begun at the same time. Equally important, doing a permanent section allows the pathologist as much time as needed to arrive at an unrushed and accurate evaluation of your tumor. If the diagnosis of cancer is made, it gives you time for a second opinion, if you wish.

It was once felt that a breast tumor was an emergency; surgery, if necessary, had to be done as quickly as possible before the tumor cells had additional time to seed to other organs. This is no longer believed to be necessary. In truth, before they can be palpated, most breast cancers have been present for a long time (in some cases, many years). A delay of a week or two will make no difference in a patient's long-term survival or well-being.

When cancer has been found, various tests are done during the interval between the biopsy and further definitive treatment, to determine if the cancer has spread beyond the breast or if it is localized to the breast alone. Testing involves x-rays, blood tests, body scans, and urinalysis. Later, when surgery is done, the axillary lymph nodes will be examined for any signs of cancer cells. Knowing the extent of involvement beyond the breast, if any, is important because it helps determine the appropriate treatment for your individual situation.

Having this time also allows you to be involved in making the decision about your own treatment and can help you feel you still have control over your body and your life. This is very important because many women, when facing cancer, feel that events in their lives are "running away with them" and that they no longer have control over their own destinies. Feeling you have some control over what will happen may be a crucial factor in determining your attitude about your disease and may influence the way you cope with the diagnosis of cancer, both before and after surgery.

According to an American Cancer Society survey of women's preferences concerning biopsy and having treatment at a later date, the following statistics emerged:

- One out of five women said they would want to consult with another doctor and get a second opinion if, as a result of the biopsy, their physician recommended a mastectomy.
- One out of three women said they would want to discuss their treatment options after the biopsy and that they would then return to surgery if it was necessary.

Perhaps most important is that this interval allows you sufficient time to learn as much as you can about your various treatment options. Today there are more than ever before, and you should know them. Gone are the days when a surgeon made all the decisions for the patient. Not every woman has *every* treatment choice (we will discuss this in Chapter 6), but you should know which choices would be realistic and reasonable for you. Knowing your medical situation along with your treatment choices, and taking the time to discuss them with your doctor, will allow you to make a realistic and informed treatment decision based on your medical and psychological needs.

The Hormone-Receptor Assay

If a biopsy indicates that your tumor is cancerous, a hormone-receptor assay test should be done to determine whether a particular cancer's growth is affected by the hormones estrogen and progesterone. The test requires a certain amount of tumor tissue to be removed and assayed. If the original biopsy is extensive enough to provide sufficient tumor tissue, the test may be done then, although it is usually done when the definitive breast surgery is performed and the entire tumor is removed. The test requires trained personnel and special equipment that is not yet widely available.

If you are scheduled for a breast tumor biopsy, you should ask your physician about this test so the appropriate arrangements can be made.

About one-third of primary breast tumors are very estrogen-dependent. Another one-third are somewhat influenced by circulating estrogens. The hormone-receptor assay test is important because there is always a possibility that the primary tumor may have already metastasized to other parts of your body. If these metastases form secondary tumors in other organs, it is helpful to know if the original tumor thrived on estrogen and progesterone. If it did, any secondary tumors appearing at a later time may be forced to shrink and even disappear if they are deprived of these hormones.

There are a number of ways to rid the circulation of these hormones if a hormone-dependent secondary tumor later appears. The ovaries can be removed surgically or by radiation treatments. Other glands, the adrenal and the pituitary, which regulate these hormones, can be manipulated. Recently, a new drug called Tamoxifen™ has been developed that inhibits the effects of circulating estrogens so another round of surgery or radiation to remove the ovaries or adrenals may be unnecessary.

Your Emotional Situation

Finding a breast lump, having a biopsy done, and then waiting for a definitive diagnosis can be agonizing. Some women feel a profound sense of dread, impending doom, and anticipatory anxiety. Others may be frightened and become convinced they have cancer and are about to die. It is difficult to imagine any woman discovering a breast lump or abnormal change without having some feelings of dread, anxiety, and even depression.

❧ Pam Reimer was a woman whose reaction to finding a breast lump and having it diagnosed was similar to many we have seen. She was a 38-year-old legal secretary, wife, and the mother of an 11-year-old son. She was a tall and statuesque woman, who dressed attractively and wore makeup with a sophisticated flair. One day, about a year earlier, while applying suntan lotion, she discovered a lump in her left breast.

She was disbelieving at first and felt the lump again and again, wondering how long it had been present. She was especially concerned because two good friends within the previous 18 months had developed breast cancer, and this disease was very much on her mind.

"My God! I thought, *me* too!" Pam said in an interview one year after her treatment for breast cancer. "I made an appointment to see my doctor the next day. It was very strange sitting in the office and waiting to be examined. I had this weird feeling that things were happening too fast, like I was living in some crazy dream world, that things were somehow unreal. Looking back on it all now, I think I knew earlier that something was wrong with my left breast. I may have known weeks and weeks before, but I blocked it out of my mind. I just dreaded the doctor examining me. I dreaded that and the thought that he would say something like, 'It's cancer.' But what could I do?

"I thought about my husband and my son—I hadn't told John yet—it didn't make any sense because I didn't know what I had. But I had this suspicion. I guess it was based on what had happened to my friends."

Pam's physician felt that further tests were warranted. A mammogram was done. It indicated a solid tumor, most likely a cancer.

"I came home that day knowing I had it, that from that

point on my life would be different, that everything was suddenly changing. I had this awful feeling . . . I can't really describe it. I felt overwhelmed, but there was this incredibly strong feeling that everything was about to spin out of control, that I wouldn't be able to keep the lid on things. That's when I told John."

Pam's husband listened carefully and immediately became involved in the diagnostic process. Pam wanted this very much. "If I'd ever had doubts about John, that maybe he didn't love me enough . . . they disappeared before this thing was over. He was fabulous! He called the doctor, and together, we made another appointment. He began reading about breast cancer and everything relating to it. He even took time off from work, sometimes, just to *be* with me."

Pam, her husband, and her surgeon agreed that she would have the biopsy done and wait for the results. They would then discuss the complete range of treatment options available in her situation.

"Those two days [between the biopsy and the results] were like I was in some kind of time warp. It was dreamlike, and I think my head was in a whirl. My husband and my brother-in-law were great . . . they stayed with me and made it as easy as they could. But there was this sense of doom everywhere.

"It's funny. I knew the minute John walked into the room the day the results came in that I had cancer. I just knew it from the way he looked, and I thought I would sink through the floor. *This is it,* I thought, and I remember thinking right there and then that I'd better start making arrangements for Danny, that all I wanted to do was to live a few more years to see him grow up . . . that's all . . . but that maybe I'd never even see him grow to be a man.

"Then it was funny . . . but do you know what I thought

about next? It wasn't that I might die, although I'd already thought about that a hundred times. I thought about my breast, that I would lose it and that I couldn't bear the thought of going through the rest of my life with only one breast! And over the next few weeks, that became the most important thing to me, that I might have to go through my life with only one breast!"

Pam, her physician, and her husband then met and discussed her tumor. They discussed its size, its location, the question about whether or not there would be "positive" nodes in her armpit, and the possibility that the disease might have spread to other organs. A complete medical work-up was begun to determine the extent of Pam's disease. All tests were normal, and it appeared so far that Pam's cancer was confined to the breast. She would have her axillary lymph nodes examined when she had her definitive surgery.

"I guess I felt a little relieved," Pam said many months later. "But still, there was the cancer, and there was the thought of losing my breast. Now, when I look back, it was the thought that I could have a new breast that helped me get through the whole thing! That seemed the most important thing to me. I never thought I was so vain, that I would value my breast as much as my life! But that's the way I felt!"

"And then I had the strangest thoughts," Pam said, laughing. "I thought about my family . . . my mother and my sisters. How come *I* had this thing? How come it was *me* and not *them?* What had *I* done that made me in some way be *singled out* for this *thing?* It's funny because I'd always felt a little left out. I mean, I'm the middle daughter and it always seemed to me that my sisters got more than I did. Always! The youngest one was a spoiled brat who couldn't take 'no' for an answer and the oldest, well, she was the *oldest,* what else can I say? But here, with cancer, *I* was the chosen one. How come? Why *me* and not one of *them?*

"Then I got angry, at everybody, I guess. But it felt strange because deep down, there was this rational part of me that kept saying, *it's crazy to be angry . . . it's nobody's fault that you've got cancer.* And yet, I felt annoyed, peeved . . . angry at my doctor, at my sisters, at my mother—did I inherit this thing from her, or from *her* mother?—and even at my husband. It was a terrible time and I sometimes wonder how I got through it. Through the first examination, the mammography, the biopsy, and then the waiting. It seemed like forever between the biopsy and the result. The result— I don't even know if that was the worst part. I was dealing with all these different feelings at one time, feelings about my life and my breasts and about all the people in my life; my husband, my son, my sisters, my mother—all of them. God! It was a terrible time!

"I even began wondering if I'd done anything to deserve this thing, this cancer, and I began thinking about guilt and punishment a lot, and about the past. Where had I gone wrong? I thought that maybe I was the only woman on earth who had these crazy thoughts about wrong and right and about what I'd done. The fact was that only a few months earlier I'd been very attracted to this man at the office, and I'd thought about what it would be like to be with him, you know . . .

"It was very strange how I tried imagining what life with one breast would be like. How would I look? What would my husband think? Would he want me . . . ever again? What about clothing? The beach? What about my idea of myself as sexy? Because I'd always had nice breasts . . .

they weren't the biggest around, but they were nicely shaped and they were nearly the perfect size for my height and weight. I always felt they were a real plus, that they made me one of the more attractive women in my group . . . my breasts and my legs."

In many ways, Pam's reaction to discovering a lump and then making arrangements for diagnosis and treatment was not at all uncommon.

Finding out you have breast cancer is traumatic for many different reasons. First there is the idea of cancer and the fear it may create: fear of death, of dying painfully, and many others. But for many women, the diagnosis of breast cancer may also mean coping with the loss of a breast, and even then, there is no guarantee the disease will not reappear at a later time.

Of course, every woman who develops breast cancer will react in her own individual way. This depends on her personality and on her life's situation—her family, her friends, how much she knows about the disease, and so on. But we see certain important themes in many of our patients. We will discuss in detail these different meanings and reactions to breast cancer in the next chapter. Here, we want to focus on coping with the diagnosis. At such a time you must deal with feelings which can flood anyone facing the physical and emotional impact of breast cancer. How do you cope with the diagnosis?

Your Surgeon and You at This Time

Your surgeon may be the most important person in determining how well you cope. If you and your doctor develop a real *rapport* and can talk about your diagnosis and treatment, you will be more able to deal with your situation over the course of the next weeks, months, and even years.

We have seen situations where a patient and a physician did not develop a good rapport. Such patients suffered greatly and became increasingly anxious and angry during their hospital stays. They became angry at the surgeon, at nurses, and at their husbands and families. They often had difficult and stormy treatments.

On the other hand, we know of many patients who have developed a "working alliance" with their surgeons and have benefited greatly from this crucial relationship. They often felt more positively about their treatments and their outlooks, and were better able to deal with various demands during this trying time in their lives.

What to Look for in Your Surgeon

Of course, you want a surgeon whose medical and surgical skills are unquestionable. But there are other important qualities you should look for because your relationship with your surgeon is going to be much more involved than the technical details of the operating room. This is true no matter what treatment method will be used—a biopsy only, a biopsy followed by minimal surgery, or a biopsy and then a possible mastectomy. Exactly what qualities make for a good rapport or working alliance between you and your surgeon?

Your surgeon should be open, communicative, and above all, honest with you. In our experience, most patients want to be told the truth about their conditions. The vast majority of patients want and need to know as much as they possibly can about their medical situations. Of course, there are some who do not wish this kind of truthfulness—who may want to know as little as possible about what is really going on and who usually let the doctor know this in some way. They use a kind of *emotional anesthesia,* which may be fine so long as it doesn't result in their pretending all is well and so long as they seek proper medical help. But for most people, the plain, solid truth is much easier to deal with than uncertainty or a murky unknown.

There are a host of myths about cancer, and these well-entrenched misconceptions make very fruitful soil for frightening fantasies and for terrifying distortions. Silence and vagueness on the part of your doctor are the last things you need in this situation. Ignorance, not-knowing, and evading the facts are your enemies! In our experience, most patients, no matter which disease they are dealing with, appreciate accurate information and a frank discussion of their treatment options. Such an approach not only helps them accept their diagnosis and situations, but also helps them work out their fears so they aren't paralyzed by irrational worries, by half-truths, or by frightening myths.

Your surgeon should tell you the exact plan for "working up" or diagnosing your breast lump. Which test(s) will be performed and why? What do they mean if the results are "positive" or "negative"? If a test indicates cancer, or a high index of suspicion of cancer, what will the next step be? Your surgeon should spend enough time with you (and your husband or another close relative, if you wish) and should answer your questions in concise, easy-to-understand terms. He or she should be willing to explain a proposed treatment plan and be willing to explain your various treatment options should the biopsy indicate cancer. (We will detail these options in Chapter 6.)

If your doctor prefers one method of treatment over others, he or she should explain why this is so and should detail the advantages of this method of treatment to you.

Your doctor should be open to the possibility of your getting a second opinion, either from another surgeon, an oncologist, or a radiotherapist.

Again, there is no need to rush. You are not in an emergency situation. Although you will require definitive treatment, it isn't imperative that it be done immediately. A cancer will not progress over the course of another week or two, so take the time you need to learn all you can and to digest what you learn about your diagnosis and any proposed treatment.

Communication with your surgeon is the key word. When this is missing, the problem may be with both the doctor and the patient. The surgeon may not have the necessary time because of a busy schedule; the patient may be upset (which is understandable) and may not know the right questions to ask.

In a sense, Pam Reimer was very lucky. She had a supportive husband who made himself an important member of the doctor-patient relationship. Also, Pam's doctor took the time to explore her treatment options with her and to make certain recommendations.

This important combination of factors helped Pam deal with this profound life crisis and with a flood of intense feelings. Pam wasn't overwhelmed by the diagnosis, although at times she *thought* things seemed strange and unreal. She sometimes *felt* like she was on a nonstop carousel that had spun out of control, but she wasn't. She and her husband absorbed the necessary information and made an intelligent and informed decision about treatment.

❦ Another patient, Carol Malone, did not fare as well. She was a 49-year-old divorced woman who was admitted to the hospital for treatment of a malignant breast lump.

Upon admission, a nurse noticed that Carol appeared fretful and depressed and made this notation in her chart.

The morning of her surgery, Carol became tearful and anxious. She told the nurse she wanted to leave the hospital as soon as possible. She had decided not to have treatment. Alarmed, the nurse sought Carol's surgeon, who spent a half hour talking with her and then called for a psychiatric consultation.

When the psychiatrist visited Carol in her room, she was already dressed and had packed her clothing. She was angry, yet tearful, and talked about how "useless" everything was. She said it would do no good to have surgery at that time. She insisted that it was likely her cancer had already spread to the rest of her body, and then she cried at length. A sense of hopelessness permeated Carol's words and even her posture as she sat in a chair at the bedside and talked. It was obvious that she was severely depressed.

Carol bemoaned being alone at that time. Her divorce had been 5 years earlier. She had no children and no relatives in New York City and felt there was no one she could count on during this crisis. "Besides," she added, "what do I have to live for?"

Carol added that she couldn't talk with her surgeon, saying he was too busy to spend time with her. The psychiatrist asked her about her treatment, and it was quickly apparent that Carol knew very little about her treatment options or about the extent of her disease. She said she felt isolated and "out of touch" with everything and could no longer tolerate the impersonal atmosphere on the ward.

The psychiatrist inquired about her family and learned that Carol had a sister living in another city. The psychiatrist then urged her to call her sister and see if it was possible to arrange for treatment there, where she would have someone she felt close to. It was clear that in her present situation Carol felt angry, alone, and victimized, by her situation and her life. A good rapport with her surgeon could have made the difference for Carol, but such a rapport requires receptive people at both ends and Carol was too upset to be able to extend herself. The stage was then set for her to feel completely overwhelmed by her circumstances and to angrily leave her surgeon, the hospital, and her treatment.

There is one other important point to be made about your relationship with your physician. It would be unrealistic to expect any surgeon to spend hours and hours with you or to give up a busy schedule to be with you exclusively even at this difficult time. Your doctor is a human being and may have some failings. Most doctors must psychologically protect themselves from becoming too personally involved with their patients, especially if they see a great many people with cancer. But what you should expect from your physician is patience, thoughtfulness, and as much information as you need to help you adjust to your diagnosis, know your treatment options, and decide on your treatment.

· FIVE ·

The Meanings
of Breast Cancer

❧

The impact of learning you have breast cancer is enormous. In our opinion, the emotional and social disruptions accompanying breast cancer are an integral part of the disease and cannot be ignored. They must be treated as seriously as the medical aspects of cancer. In fact, the many meanings of breast cancer are so crucial to women that they are profoundly influencing the ways in which the disease is now being treated. We certainly agree with the physician who, in a January 1984 *New York* magazine article, was quoted as saying: "Around every lesion there happens to be a human being."

Anyone who has ever been touched by breast cancer knows that intense and complex emotional issues come to the fore with this disease. While our comments in this chapter cannot be applied to every woman, because people react individually to this life crisis, we frequently see the same vital concerns in our patients. These issues cannot be underestimated since they will influence a woman's adjustment to her diagnosis, her compliance with her treatment, and her entire well-being.

Cancer and Fear

The large group of diseases called cancer is the scourge of our time. Much like tuberculosis and pneumonia in the nineteenth century, cancer conjures up great fear. Fear is always more devastating and intense when there are few answers and when the unknown looms before us. As more knowledge about cancer is slowly pieced together, success stories in the treatment of cancer are becoming more common. Yet somehow, we hear very little about these steps of progress. Understandably, people focus on the unknown, perhaps because it is so awesome and fearful. The possibility of death and dying seem to leave a much greater mark than progress without absolute answers.

To some extent, the public perception of cancer is a result of the various media giving the disease a great deal of exposure and prominence. Hardly a day goes by without reports about cancer-inducing chemicals such as Agent Orange, insecticides, toxic wastes, certain food preservatives, and a variety of other substances found in everyday life, or without the obituary of some prominent person who died of cancer.

Awareness of cancer is also heightened partly because today, Americans are living longer. Generally, cancer tends to be a disease of older people, so more people than ever before are developing cancers of all types. This does not necessarily indicate an increase in the incidence of these diseases; it simply means there are more older people and more sophisticated methods of detecting these diseases.

Amidst such heightened awareness of cancer, it is no wonder that most women react to the news that they have breast cancer with intense and sometimes overwhelming feelings and thoughts.

Of course, the diagnosis of cancer of any kind can arouse

many profound fears in anyone—fear of the unknown, fear of what the disease may lead to, fear about how one's life may be changed, fear about death and the *way* one may die, or fear of chronic and painful disability. But for a woman, in addition to these fears, breast cancer is unique because it arouses many concerns about the loss of a breast. This can have profound meanings for any woman.

❧ Self-preservation is not always a woman's primary concern. Carol Collins was 40 years old when she discovered a lump in her breast. She was a successful marketing analyst for a large corporation and was leading a good life. She discovered her lump early, and yet, assumed that her prognosis would be dim. After the diagnosis was made, she left her job convinced she would die shortly. Her major worry was about her 12-year-old son, Paul, whom she and her husband had adopted some years earlier.

"I couldn't stop thinking about Paul. I kept thinking, *I'm going to die . . . that's no tragedy, but what about Paul?* I kept thinking that somehow, it was all my fault, that I should have done things differently. Don't ask me what. But here I was, with cancer. And we'd tried so long to have a child and we couldn't. You can't imagine the trouble we went through, the absolute craziness we went through to finally adopt a child. I was so desperate I'd have taken *any* child, any age, any color. Anything. And now, what's going to happen to him? He won't have a mother. Somehow, I just feel I failed. Completely."

Another deeply disturbing concern for many women, no matter how early a cancer is detected, is that they must contend with the possibility that there may be a recurrence of a potentially fatal disease.

🌿 Barbara Conti, who detected her breast lump early, had a mastectomy and was symptom-free for 12 years before being evaluated for a breast reconstruction. Nevertheless, she admitted the impact her disease had had on her life:

"You know, it's not that I don't think about it, about the possibility that it might come back. I do. I'd like to forget it, but I can't. Not really.

"Sometimes, when things are going very well—when I'm really happy with my life, with my husband and the kids, and when I know I've got lots to be thankful for . . . well, sometimes I just see that scar and I'm reminded about cancer. It almost whispers in my ear: *cancer* . . .

"Then, a little quiver goes through me and I get this strange feeling. I usually put it out of my mind. It's not like the first year or two after the mastectomy where if I had the slightest sniffle or a backache or something, that I had this horrible thought: *It's the cancer!* That's gone now. But there's that little whisper every now and then. Maybe that's why I want reconstruction—just so I won't have this scar and maybe I won't be reminded of it so easily. But no matter what, the thought never goes away."

The truth is that any woman who has breast cancer, no matter how successful the treatment or how many years later she is alive and well, must face the ever-present knowledge that she has had and may still have a potentially fatal disease. Breast cancer is a life crisis, and for any woman, it will require previously untapped energies and emotional resources.

Concerns about the physical consequences of cancer, about dying or disability, or about chronic pain and suffering are, of course, not limited to the patient herself. The diagnosis of breast cancer has a profound impact on a woman's family.

We will go more into detail about the family and its reaction to the disease in Chapter 9.

The Loss of a Breast

As we've said, breast cancer is traumatic not only because of fears it may arouse about death and dying but because it may involve the loss of a breast. These concerns are so great that today much of the controversy about the best method of treatment for breast cancer is based on cosmetic considerations. Only in recent years has the medical community begun to appreciate the meanings that a woman's breasts have for her and the profound feelings that breast loss may arouse.

Some years ago, if a woman voiced feelings about saving her breast, she would have felt she was being vain or neurotic. The prevailing sentiment seemed to be, *You're getting away with your life. Be thankful! Don't worry about something as trivial as a breast!* Today, more and more emphasis is placed on a woman's reaction to the possibility of breast loss and to her alternatives in treating breast cancer. We will have much more to say about this later. At this point we will simply say that today, with less extensive surgery, with radiation, and with new breast reconstruction techniques, there is no need for a woman who has been treated for breast cancer to feel irreversibly mutilated.

There can be no doubt that many women believe the size and shape of their breasts are one of the primary determinants of their attractiveness. Recent social trends may have lessened the traditional emphasis on breasts (even on a woman's looks) as having such importance, but it is difficult to say that women will someday be evaluated less on their physical attributes and more on other qualities.

However, these are broad social issues. We must concern ourselves with the *individual* woman who, when encountering breast cancer, must deal with the traumatic impact of the disease, not only on her life expectancy but on her looks and on her entire *image* of herself.

If a woman has been conditioned to think of herself as being basically worthwhile because of certain physical attributes, then the possible loss of a breast threatens a fundamental component of her entire sense of herself.

Recall Pam Reimer who, when breast cancer was diagnosed, *became as worried about the thought of losing her breast* as she was about the possibility that she had a potentially fatal disease.

"I couldn't bear going through the rest of my life with only one breast!" she said during an interview many months after her surgery.

"Now, when I look back, it was the thought that I could have a new breast that helped me get through the whole thing! That seemed the most important thing to me . . . that I could get a new breast. I never thought I was so vain, that I would value my breast as much as my life. But that's the way I felt."

Pam's thoughts and feelings were not unique. Her sense of herself as a woman and her measure of herself as a person were threatened. And then, too, her entire self-image was on the line. She had always valued having good-looking legs and breasts and felt these attributes made her one of the more attractive women in her group. No wonder the threat of losing a breast was so horrifying to her. Her breasts were significant components of her entire view of herself and of her self-esteem. If a woman feels this way, then the loss of a breast will be extremely meaningful.

Then, too, breasts are psychologically, and realistically, equated with *motherhood,* with nurturing and with general well-being. The threat of breast loss strikes at this basic self-image and the woman facing such a possibility may find herself doubting her worth as a woman and as a mother.

Finally, the loss of *any* body part threatens one's entire concept of the *whole* self as an integrated, functioning, and healthy person. A loss of any part of the "self" can make a person feel lessened or devalued, especially if the lost part is viewed by so many people as being an integral component of one's attractiveness, sexuality, and wholeness as a woman, a wife, and a mother. The loss of a breast can make a woman begin to doubt she will ever be sexually desirable.

🌿 Barbara Conti had a great deal to say about how she viewed herself.

"I suppose that after a while I got used to it, because I wonder why I've waited so long to look into reconstruction. But there was a period of time when I was obsessed with breasts—with large, round breasts, the kind that stick out to here," she said with a laugh as she held her arms out from her chest.

"There was this day, a few months after my mastectomy . . . well, up 'til then I'd thought my husband would never want me again, that I was a freak of some kind. But on this particular day, things were going better. I think it was about four months later, and I actually felt I *wanted to be good to myself,* to give myself a treat.

"I found myself in Bloomingdale's, in one of the dress departments, and I picked out this lovely dress—of course there could be no low neckline—and I got into the dressing booth and began changing. I felt I might finally begin seeing myself as attractive again, and it felt really good.

"Well, as I was getting into this dress, I adjusted my bra, and my prosthesis slipped out onto the floor. It rolled away from me and went under the partition—into the next booth! I knew there was another woman in there, and for a second, I didn't know what to do. I was frozen. It seemed like the world would end. Then I guess I reacted without thinking . . . it was automatic.

"The next thing I knew I was out of the booth and I opened the other door. Without looking, I bent down and picked it up. I guess I mumbled something apologetic, and I rushed out. Then, I don't even remember how, I found myself back in my own dress with my coat on, out on Lexington Avenue in the middle of all those people. Tears were running down my cheeks and I felt like the most humiliated and worthless woman on the face of the earth. I can't remember anything worse than that day and those feelings."

Certainly such feelings can run the gamut from hope to despair, to a sense of being incomplete, frightened, and inadequate. The medical community has been slow to appreciate the profound feelings breast cancer and breast loss can arouse in women. It took years to develop alternatives for women who were devastated by having a breast amputated. Such a lack of responsiveness to women's concerns has understandably led to a certain amount of resentment and even anger at physicians. Increasingly over the last few years, more and more women have asked the question, "If cancer of the penis were as common as cancer of the breast, would alternatives to radical surgery have been developed much earlier? Would reconstruction have been placed on the back burner for as long as it has been?"

Today, a great deal of consideration is being given to

the psychological meanings of the breast, to the trauma of breast loss, and to the concerns women have about disfigurement. These issues figure prominently in the controversies going on in medical circles about the "best" method of treating certain breast cancers.

Many physicians have been surprised to realize that older women have the same concerns about their breasts and the possibility of disfigurement as younger women do. Feeling whole, feeling one is attractive and completely defined as a woman, a wife, and a mother, are not solely the feelings of younger women.

Some older women have felt guilty when, after losing a breast, they longed to see themselves as attractive and sexually alluring once again. The breast loss had reawakened awareness of their own sexuality and of the meanings of their breasts. The prevailing sentiment for some women could be, *I'm too old for these feelings; I should be ashamed of myself.* Because of these feelings, some older women would hesitate seeking breast reconstruction for fear of appearing vain or overly concerned with sexual or cosmetic concerns. Today, this situation is beginning to change, especially as the general public and medical community become more aware of the sexual needs and self-esteem concerns of older people.

Other Feelings

At some point when dealing with breast cancer in herself, nearly every woman affected will feel angry. Such feelings may begin as a sense of injustice, which can then lead to feeling outraged. Recall how Pam Reimer felt when the diagnosis of breast cancer was made. She was the middle of three daughters and felt that in all other things, her sisters had gotten more than she had. "But there, with cancer, *I* was the chosen one. How come? Why *me* and not one of *them?*" she asked with an angry tone to her voice.

Some patients may feel angry at nearly everyone, especially people in the medical profession. "Why isn't there a cure for breast cancer?" the patient may ask angrily, and her hostility may focus on the nearest and most convenient targets: nurses, physicians, a social worker, or her own family. Other patients may express a sense of disappointment and then anger at "fate" or anger at God. Much of this stems from a feeling of having been betrayed by "fate," by God, and by one's own body.

Guilt is a feeling that is rarely rational when it surfaces in relation to illness, especially in breast cancer. Pam Reimer wondered aloud about her having been attracted to a man at the office. Perhaps, she imagined, she had brought on the cancer. It is very common for patients to imagine they are being punished for some real or imagined misdeed, whether it was in thought or action.

❧ "I know this sounds crazy," Barbara Conti said, "and I know it's not really true, but I sometimes find myself wondering if maybe the fact that I used to prefer foreplay, that my right breast was very sensitive—the nipple—and I found it very exciting with my husband. Maybe that had something to do with cancer."

Barbara Conti's thoughts, like so many other women's facing breast cancer, found a focus on some "sin" or "flaw" in the fabric of her life; one which she imagined could be the possible cause of her disease. "Pinning" the cause of the disease on some imagined misdeed is, among other things, an attempt to understand what is happening, to bring order out of chaos and to somehow gain control over the frightening feelings cancer can arouse.

❦ Guilt can take other forms as well. Lucille Greene, a woman who developed breast cancer at the age of 53, was also worried that her daughter (19 years old at the time of Lucille's mastectomy) might someday develop breast cancer.

"I know these things can be passed on through the genes, that my daughter runs a higher-than-average risk of getting breast cancer. And I guess in some way I feel a little guilty about that, as though it's my fault. I even wonder if she thinks about it, and that maybe she's angry with me."

The many strong feelings that breast cancer arouses may cause some patients to deny they are seriously ill. Some psychiatrists feel that denial is necessary and even healthy for certain women who are overwhelmed when the disease is first diagnosed. For them, denial may become an emotional anesthetic. Then, as time passes and the threat lessens—which often happens when a woman learns the *facts* of her situation rather than feeling overcome by fantasies—the reality can be absorbed. Then, the disease with its problems and challenges may be faced.

The fears, anxieties, and worries any woman can have about breast cancer are intensely personal and profound, but they are absolutely normal worries. They are the emergency reactions of every patient we have seen when facing the unknown and spring from a very basic sense of survival. Only when such feelings are too intense and get out of hand are they working against you. When you recognize them and understand their meanings you can harness them and mobilize yourself into a plan of action that can help you have the best outlook possible.

The figures today are very clear. Breast cancer is not an automatic death sentence nor is it an automatic prescription for mutilation. Women whose breast cancers are detected early have an excellent chance of surviving for years to come, and they may also avoid lifelong disfigurement.

Your greatest assets in facing breast cancer are knowing all you can about it and knowing about today's treatment options. Then you will be less likely to be overwhelmed by fears and by feelings of helplessness.

Frequently Asked Questions

I'm a 46-year-old woman and recently had a lump biopsied. The diagnosis was cancer. I'm in the middle of many hospital tests now, and I have all these morbid thoughts. What can I do?

The period of time following the diagnosis of breast cancer is difficult for any woman and her family. There may be a torrent of morbid thoughts as well as hopeful ones; there is often fear, anxiety, depression, hopelessness, despair, anger, and most of all, shock when the diagnosis comes. While every woman reacts differently, there are certain thoughts and feelings we see very often when the diagnosis of breast cancer is made. You are going through some of these feelings at the present time.

Your tests are to evaluate the extent of the disease and tell if the cancer has spread beyond your breast. Your outlook will depend on what these tests indicate. But no matter how good the outlook may be, it would be unusual for you not to have thoughts about death and dying. After all, cancer conjures up so many horrible images for most people. Often, these images have little to do with the reality of a given situation.

Do not be surprised if at this time, right after the diagnosis, you have many conflicting thoughts and feelings. Many women report that the time they learned their diagnoses was the most difficult. Here is where you need the support and help of your family, and here too is where you need the facts of your case explained in a clear and honest way by your physician. Once you know these facts, you will be better able to realistically deal with your situation. You will be less likely to be deluged by morbid thoughts, many of which may be fantasy.

I'm 39 years old. I've just been told that my biopsy was positive and that I have breast cancer. My doctor says the prognosis is probably very good because the tests show that my tumor is very small and there is no evidence that it has reached any other parts of my body. The lymph node surgery hasn't been done yet. I have two children, ages 10 and 13. Should I tell them?

Yes. This is not a time for secrets or for withholding the truth. You need the support and understanding of your entire family. Equally important, your children will want and need to know exactly what is going on. They will pick up on many cues and signals and will know something is "wrong" anyway. It will benefit everyone concerned if the facts are honestly out in the open. This will allow everyone to cope with what's going on. Breast cancer is a family crisis, and if circumstances permit, you should share what you know with your family.

I'm 49 years old and my breast biopsy has come back "positive." I know at some point I'll have to tell my husband, because I'm going to have a mastectomy in two weeks. But I'm not sure he'll be able to deal with this. What should I do?

Your husband is your partner in life, and as such, he would want to share this difficult burden with you. Imagine how left out and possibly resentful he might feel when he finds out later. He may feel that you didn't trust him or that you didn't think he could cope. You may decide not to tell other people about your breast cancer, but your husband is the one person who needs to know and who, most likely, would want to know about your situation. Unless there are very compelling reasons for you to withhold this crucially important information from him, you are best off telling him exactly what is going on. He may surprise you not only with his ability to cope but with his capacity to be supportive in ways you have never before imagined.

My wife is 42 years old. She just had a biopsy of a breast lump, which came back as cancer. Her doctor has recommended a course of treatment, but she seems to want nothing to do with it. She says things will be whatever they will be, and she wants to go on as though nothing is wrong. What can I do?

This kind of fatalism can be dangerous. Certainly, your wife should undergo a reasonable course of treatment if it is recommended. Her wish to leave everything to fate could possibly result in an untreated disease with grave consequences. It is understandable that you may be frustrated and worried, even angry, especially if the doctor indicates that her prognosis is a good one if she receives treatment. You must be forceful and persistent in this, and you must feel confident you know what is best for her and the family at this point. You may have to engineer her treatment because she's using denial and a fatalistic sense of complacency in a way that could prove dangerous for her.

You must give her the facts and you must encourage her physician to tell her exactly *why* this course of treatment is recommended and what the consequences may be if treatment is *not* pursued. The best way to fight her fatalism is with facts that will be a convincing argument in favor of treatment. You may actually have to be somewhat manipulative here, letting your wife know that the best way she can show her love for you is to get the proper treatment for her disease. Also, psychological counseling may be very helpful.

I'm in my early 40s. I've been divorced for a number of years, and I've recently learned I have breast cancer. When I think about it, I don't seem to care too much. I feel I have nothing to live for. Can you help me?

First, you have asked if you can be helped, so, despite your depression, there is some wish to get on with your life and to have a meaningful future. You are dealing with two very loaded emotional issues: divorce and cancer. This has led you into a depression. Depression often follows a meaningful life loss. It may be the loss of someone you love (through divorce or death) or the loss of something vital to you (your health or a job). But before we can talk more about your depression, we must make certain that you are going to get the proper treatment for your disease. We may not have 6 months in which to explore your problems right now; you must mobilize yourself and get treatment for your breast cancer. That's the primary issue at this moment.

It seems that your previous loss (your marriage) has left you in a position where you don't have sufficient emotional support or closeness in your life right now. This may have left you depressed enough not to pursue your treatment options for the breast cancer. And the cancer has been another blow to your already sagging self-esteem. You must get treatment as soon as possible!

You make it clear that you are dealing with *feelings* more than with facts; that you *feel* there is nothing to live for. But remember, making the decision not to seek treatment may have permanent consequences, and you should not make such a decision while you are in a *temporary* frame of mind.

Your depression may lift quickly with the proper psychological treatment. You would probably find counseling with a psychiatrist helpful, and you might possibly benefit from a course of antidepressant medication.

My wife has just received the results of a breast biopsy. It's cancer. But she has no reaction at all! I've been upset and crying, but she's as calm as can be. Am I overreacting? Or should I try to bring out some of these feelings from within her?

It's very difficult to ascertain whether you're overreacting. You certainly can be upset; after all, none of this is good news. But what are the facts of your wife's case? What has her physician said about her disease and its treatment? These are crucial points to consider. We have seen some husbands overreact, and in certain cases, a husband may be preoccupied about what may happen to *him* if he loses his wife. Some husbands begin imagining it's inevitable that their wife will die, and they become frightened. This can result in overcompensation, with fretting and worrying and a kind of smothering solicitousness.

As for your wife's reaction, it's difficult to know how she

should react to the diagnosis. She may have many thoughts and feelings about all this, and no doubt they will surface in time. Right now, she may need some kind of emotional or psychic anesthesia to keep these frightening thoughts to a minimum. The important thing is that she's not pretending everything is fine. She is apparently seeking the appropriate medical help, so she's not ignoring her condition to her detriment.

As for bringing out some of your wife's feelings at this time, it is probably not a good idea. You cannot force-feed feelings to someone. It's quite likely that she will express herself as time goes by.

I'm 41 years old. There's a lot of breast cancer in my family, and I have lumpy breasts. I've had one breast biopsy done— it was negative. I constantly worry about breast cancer, and I'm tired of running to doctors. What can be done to help me?

You are in the high-risk group of women for developing breast cancer. However, as we mentioned in Chapter 2, the statistics become much less meaningful when applied to any one individual woman at any particular time in her life.

It's understandable that you may be worried about this. You should practice BSE regularly each month, and should seriously consider having a low-dose mammogram taken each year. In addition, you should also consider seeing your physician twice each year for a thorough breast examination.

You may have become so concerned about the *possibility* of developing breast cancer that your worry has begun eroding into other areas of your and your family's life. If this is so, you may have developed *cancerphobia:* an irrational fear of the disease coupled with the conviction that the least significant thing—a sore, some ache or pain somewhere in the body—may indicate cancer. If these feelings persist (and if they compromise other areas of your life) you may wish to consider psychological counseling. Once this is explored, if you still fear developing breast cancer, you may consider a subcutaneous mastectomy with reconstruction (see Chapter 6).

I've recently had the diagnosis made of breast cancer. I will be going into the hospital next week. I've told my best friend, and it's become clear to me that she's shying away from me. This is a very turbulent time for me and I'd hoped I could depend on her, but I now feel hurt and abandoned. Is there anything I can do?

When the diagnosis of breast cancer is made, many people are affected. Your family and your friends (if you tell them) will react in different ways. Even the word *cancer* conjures up a variety of thoughts and feelings. For each person involved, there is the dilemma of how to react and of what to do. While we will talk more about these situations in a later chapter, it is important to mention some of these difficulties now.

Your friend may not know how to react to your news. Many people are uncomfortable with someone who has cancer; they don't know what to say or do for fear of appearing either insensitive or patronizing. Some friends may tell you, "Everything will be fine. You're all right; don't worry," and they may appear supportive and concerned. However, we've seen women who have felt that such "support" and "reassurance" is patronizing and trivializes a real-life crisis through which they were going.

On the other hand, some friends may feel very threatened by your condition. This may be totally irrational, as when someone harbors the fantasy that cancer is contagious, or that a person with cancer is somehow "repulsive" or to be avoided. Or people can simply be threatened by their feeling uncomfortable with someone who has the disease. This may be what's happening with your friend.

Try not to be too harsh in judging your friend. She may need time to come to terms with her own complex feelings about you, about cancer, about what the disease means to her, rationally and irrationally, and about many other things. Try remembering what it was like when a good friend's spouse or parent died; recall how helpless you felt at trying to be consoling and recall how hollow your words of support and solace may have sounded in your own ears.

Of course, your having breast cancer is not the same as someone's losing a spouse or a parent; there is no death sentence here. But people may be dealing with the same *feelings,* and often, feelings are more important in determining how we react than are facts. Give yourself and your friend time to adjust to all that has happened in your life.

SIX

It's Cancer—What Next?

❦

There are two important areas to consider when treating breast cancer. The first is the *local or regional disease,* which involves the breast lump itself and the lymph nodes that drain that area. The second is the patient's *overall body,* if the cancer cells have spread beyond the local area. Surgery and radiation (separately or combined) are used to treat local breast and lymph node disease. Chemotherapy and hormone therapy are used if cancer cells have spread to the body in general.

Some patients have cancer confined to the breast only. Others may also have malignant cells that have spread to other parts of the body. Depending on how far the disease has progressed at the time it is diagnosed, different treatment methods may be used. In our view, the decision about which treatment method should be used demands the cooperation of experts who should function as a team.

In treating any patient for breast cancer, many things must be considered. The tumor must be assessed. The regional lymph nodes must be examined. So must the rest of the body be examined to see if tumor cells have spread beyond the breast and lymph nodes. Also, any breast tissue left behind after treatment must be considered for the possibility of recurrence. And after all this has been considered, there is still the *person:* her psychological and cosmetic concerns must be taken into account and treated.

Right now, we are still learning a great deal about breast cancer and how best to treat it. Studies are underway in all areas of breast cancer treatment, and some researchers feel important answers are just around the corner. It is especially necessary at a time like this for the patient to benefit from close *teamwork* among specialists from all areas. Through the sharing of the latest insights between these experts, a sound treatment plan can be offered to any patient. We will detail this approach later in this chapter.

If your biopsy comes back "positive" for cancer, the most important thing to remember is that you must remain calm and clear-thinking. You have *not* been handed a death sentence! You are facing a life crisis, but there are ways you can deal with it.

Comparing yourself with someone you know who had breast cancer is unfair to yourself, since there are many different "types" of breast cancer. You must learn about *your* breast cancer and the extent to which it affects your breast (the local disease), the extent, if any, to which it has spread to the lymph nodes (regional disease), and the extent, if any, to which it may have spread to other parts of your body.

Also remember that different women vary in their response to cancer and to treatment. Some have a more effective system of natural defense than others. The course of breast cancer is affected by many things: your general health, the involvement or noninvolvement of lymph nodes and other organs, and your tumor's sensitivity to your body's hormones.

Knowing all this will help you ask the proper questions when you discuss your situation with your doctor. Don't be intimidated or frightened. You can learn much more about your disease than you think possible.

After your biopsy and diagnosis, an attempt should be made to learn if the disease is local—confined to the breast— or if it is systemic—having spread beyond the breast to your system at large. The proper treatment will depend upon the extent to which the disease has progressed. To determine this, certain medical tests must be done.

These tests should include an assessment of the biopsied tumor (its size, position, and type) and your doctor's assessment by physical examination of whether the cancer has spread to the axillary lymph nodes. Later, during surgery, a sample of these same lymph nodes will be taken to determine this microscopically.

The tests usually done to determine if breast cancer has spread beyond the local area of the breast are:

- A mammogram of both breasts. In some cases, when a cancer is found, there are other cancerous lesions in that breast or in the opposite breast, though they have not yet been detected. This points out the multicentric or multifocal nature of breast cancer. It may arise from many different areas within the tissue of either breast. The mammogram may also be used as a baseline study when looking for any possible future changes in your other breast.
- Blood tests to determine if other organs have been affected by the cancer.
- X-rays and scans. X-rays of the ribs and the lungs will

detect if cancer cells have spread to these areas. Scans of various organs such as the liver or the bones are done by injecting a radioactive substance into the body. This material will collect in any cancerous tissue. A special camera will pick up this contrast.

Why It Is Important to Determine if the Lymph Nodes Are Involved

Determining the extent of the cancer's spread, if any, to the regional lymph nodes is all-important in assessing any patient's probable outcome. Breast cancer cells may spread in several ways. They may extend directly into nearby tissues. This may happen if the cancer cells are left behind when a breast tumor is removed. They may escape into the bloodstream and travel to other areas of the body. Or they may flow into the lymphatic system, where they then meet the axillary and internal mammary lymph nodes.

At these nodes, the cancer cells encounter the important first line of the body's defense system, special white cells that can attack and destroy them. This ability, as well as the number of invading cancer cells, may vary from patient to patient. If the immune system is healthy and strong and the number of tumor cells is small, the white cells may be able to eliminate the threat of the cancer spreading. Sometimes, however, the number of cancer cells may be great, and the patient's immune system may be weakened and not do a good job in fighting off and destroying them.

Physicians have recently become aware that when cancer cells are found in the lymph nodes, it may mean that they have also gone *beyond* this line of the body's defense to other parts of the body. These tumor cells may or may not flourish and form secondary tumors elsewhere.

What we are saying is this: The single most important

predictor of prognosis for breast cancer is the determination of whether or not the axillary lymph nodes are involved with tumor cells. Statistics bear this out. There is a very high cure rate when a small tumor is detected early, and before the axillary lymph nodes are involved with cancer— when the nodes are "negative" for cancer cells. The survival rate drops when the axillary lymph nodes are "positive," or involved with cancer cells. This is why it is crucial for the surgeon to take a sample of the axillary lymph nodes at the time of surgery.

From this discussion it should be clear that physicians may not always be aiming for a total cure in treating breast cancer. For a patient with extensive involvement of the regional lymph nodes and metastases, the objective is to extend the patient's survival as long as possible. For a woman who has *only* local disease, confined to the breast with the lymph nodes not involved, the physician's aim is to *cure* the disease. This again emphasizes the importance of early detection.

After the surgery is performed and the axillary lymph nodes are examined, this data, together with the preoperative test results, is used to "stage" the disease. The stage of any breast cancer is a good predictor of your outlook and your treatment choices. Here are the stages of breast cancer:

Stage I. A tumor less than 2 centimeters in diameter. There is no evidence of spread to the lymph nodes and no evidence of metastasis to other organs. In other words, the disease is local; it is limited to the breast only.

Stage II. A tumor between 2 and 5 centimeters in diameter. There may be some spread of tumor cells to as many as four lymph nodes but there is no evidence of metastasis to other organs.

Stage III. A tumor larger than 5 centimeters. The nodes are more involved and may have become fixed to each other.

There is no evidence of spread to more distant organs.

Stage IV. A tumor that has spread, often locally, with extension to the chest wall and skin. In addition to the regional lymph node involvement, the cancer has spread to other parts of the body as determined by the various preoperative tests (bone scan, x-rays, blood tests, and so forth).

Treatment of the Local and Regional Disease

There is a great deal of discussion today about the use of surgery and radiation to treat local and regional breast cancer. The public is now aware that surgery that is less extensive than the radical mastectomy is available, and more attempts are being made to either save the breast or provide less disfiguring alternatives without compromising the attempt to eradicate disease. There has been a good deal of controversy both within and outside the medical community. Some discussions pit surgeons against radiotherapists and split the treatment of local and regional breast cancer into separate "camps," each adhering to one treatment method. Many women have found themselves confused by the range of treatment options. Even more distressing to some has been the problem of physician bias where some doctors, favoring one specific treatment method, have "steered" their patients in the direction of such treatment.

In the following sections, the various methods of treating local and regional breast cancer by surgery and radiation either separately or in combination are discussed. We will also explain how to ensure an unbiased and thorough investigation of your treatment options. Once you are aware of these options, you can intelligently discuss them with your doctors and then decide which treatment is best suited for your needs.

Surgery Alone

THE HALSTED RADICAL MASTECTOMY

Surgery was first used to treat breast cancer in the late nineteenth century. Because of the prevailing social and psychological influences of the day—modesty about self-examination or about a woman baring her body, even to a physician—and because of a heavy dose of ignorance about this disease, women who finally came for treatment often had extraordinarily large breast tumors. The radical mastectomy was first done in 1894 by Dr. William S. Halsted, an American surgeon practicing at Johns Hopkins Medical Center in Baltimore. This operation became the most commonly used procedure for treating breast cancer.

It involves removing the entire breast, the skin, the pectoral muscles, and the axillary lymph nodes. Such an extensive procedure was used because of the size of the tumors being seen at the time and because it was believed that breast cancer was strictly a local disease of the breast. Therefore, the thinking went, all the diseased tissue had to be removed along with a border of normal tissue.

Until recently, the Halsted radical mastectomy was the treatment given to most women with breast cancer, no matter how large or small the tumor. However, there were serious aftereffects of this operation. Removal of the lymph nodes resulted in poor lymphatic drainage, which caused swelling of the arm on the side of the operation. Removal of the pectoral muscles caused severe limitation of motion of that arm and stiffness of the shoulder. In addition, the absence of the pectoral muscles created a sunken chest wall, which was quite disfiguring.

By the early 1950s, some surgeons began attempting to reduce the debilitating afteraffects of the radical mastectomy by modifying the operation and removing less tissue. When it was seen that the 5-year survival rates (the percentage of people alive 5 years after the treatment, the traditional measure of success when combating cancer) and the recurrence rates with less extensive surgery were comparable to those of the Halsted operation, more physicians slowly began abandoning the more radical procedure. As a result, it is not frequently performed today. There are certain situations, however, when because of the size and position of the tumor, a radical operation may be required.

MODIFIED RADICAL MASTECTOMY

Throughout the 1960s and 1970s, increasing numbers of surgeons performed less extensive surgery when treating breast cancer. By 1982, the modified radical mastectomy was the procedure used in three-quarters of all surgery performed in the United States for breast cancer. It has become the standard treatment against which other treatment methods have been measured.

The modified radical mastectomy involves removing the breast, the overlying skin and nipple, fat, and most of the axillary lymph nodes. The pectoral muscles are left intact so there is no hollowness beneath the clavicle (the collarbone). With this operation, the breast may then be reconstructed at the time of surgery or later.

Surgery and Radiation Combined

Radiation may be used to shrink a very large tumor to an operable size. It may be used to control breast cancer in patients who cannot undergo surgery for medical reasons or when cancer is at a very advanced stage. Or it may be used in combination with surgery.

Radiation that affects the cell's DNA, making it incapable of replication, is effective against cancer because cells that divide very rapidly, like cancer cells, are more vulnerable to x-rays than normal cells. Thus radiation directed at cancer cells will stop them from dividing, and they will eventually die. Since normal cells are affected by radiation too, the doses and areas of treatment must be carefully calculated to minimize damage to normal tissues.

Radiotherapy is used to treat local and regional disease, not to destroy cancer cells that have spread to other parts of the body. Doctors feel the best candidates for radiation therapy are those who have early cancer confined to the breast (Stage I).

Over the years, important advances have been made in radiation technology. Older x-ray machines sometimes caused severe damage to normal cells in other organs. The newest machines direct supervoltage radiation at the treatment site and can be controlled to deliver their doses to specific depths within the body tissues, sparing underlying organs like the lungs, the heart, and the ribs. The rays penetrate the skin, barely damaging it, and can still kill cancer cells.

The following treatments combine surgery and radiation:

PARTIAL MASTECTOMY FOLLOWED BY RADIATION

Here, the tumor and 2 to 3 centimeters of surrounding tissue are removed. The breast is partially saved. It is less extensive surgery than the operations we have so far described. To kill any remaining cancer cells in the breast, radiation therapy may be given after surgery. Then, as previously mentioned, the lymph nodes must also be examined through a separate incision made in the axilla.

LUMPECTOMY (TYLECTOMY) FOLLOWED BY RADIATION

This is the least extensive surgery of all options. It removes only the tumor and a small margin of surrounding breast tissue, leaving the muscles, the skin, and the lymph nodes intact. It is less disfiguring than a mastectomy or than a partial mastectomy. Here too, to stage the disease, a separate incision is made into the axilla at the time of the lumpectomy. A portion of the regional lymph nodes is removed and examined under a microscope for evidence of tumor spread. Any lymph nodes which appear grossly suspicious or cancerous are also removed. The procedure is then followed up by radiation therapy of the breast area to kill any cancer cells that may remain behind. Because surgery is less extensive, the patient usually receives more radiotherapy following a lumpectomy than she would receive after a partial mastectomy.

If positive nodes are found in the axilla, this is presumptive evidence that cancer cells have spread beyond the local or regional area to other parts of the body. Many physicians will then recommend a course of chemotherapy to eradicate these cancer cells. This may be done after a modified radical mastectomy or after a lumpectomy.

Several studies have shown that patients with early breast cancer, if treated by lumpectomy and follow-up radiation, have survival rates as good as those who have undergone the modified radical mastectomy. Some physicians, however, do not feel these studies have been performed for a sufficient length of time to draw definite conclusions, and longer-term studies are still being conducted.

Radiotherapy Treatments

Some time after your surgery, arrangements are made for the breast to be irradiated. Before the first session, a radiotherapist marks the treatment area with indelible ink which must not be removed or washed off during the course of treatment. These markings delineate the target area so the radiation is properly placed during each session.

Most courses of radiotherapy are given over a 5- or 6-week period, 5 days each week. Each session takes 15 to 20 minutes. The correct position must be assumed beneath the radiation machine, and there may be minor adjustments and calibrations of the target area at the beginning of each session. The actual time of irradiation is about 1 minute per session.

To avoid years of exposure to x-ray scatter, the radiation therapist leaves the treatment room while beams are delivered to the patient's breast. It can seem ominous to be lying alone in a room while staring up at such awesome technology, but most patients quickly get used to the experience.

The skin and other structures can sustain only a limited amount of radiation without being damaged. This limits the total amount of x-radiation that can be delivered to the breast by the x-ray machine during the treatments. You may require additional treatment delivered internally, rather than externally by machine. The radioisotope iridium 192 (in pellet or bead form) is inserted into the remaining breast tissue, using either local or general anesthesia, at the site where the cancerous tissue was removed. This "internally delivered" treatment allows additional radiation to be safely given.

The dose needed is carefully calculated in any specific case and the implant remains in place for the necessary time. This may take 2 to 5 days. You are strictly confined to a hospital room and during this time your visitors are limited. You should not be visited by pregnant women or adolescent girls because of the possible effects of radiation on the fetus or on young, developing breast tissue. The removal of the implants marks the completion of the radiation treatment.

There are some side effects of radiation therapy, but they are usually minimal. They may include:

- Mild fatigue, which will diminish soon after the course of treatment.
- Hairline rib fractures, which occasionally occur.
- Some mild feelings of nausea, but this is fairly rare.
- Irritation of underlying lung or bronchial tissue, which is usually transient.
- Certain skin reactions at the site of the treatments. Initially there may be a sunburnlike reaction with reddening, burning, and itching. In some women, this can lead to permanent loss of color to the nipple area, a reaction which may take as long as 5 years to develop. These skin reactions are most common in fair-skinned, red-haired women. The transient itchiness, dryness, and tenderness may be alleviated with appropriate lotions and medications.

Hair loss, nausea, vomiting, and loss of appetite are side effects often associated with chemotherapy and with irradiation of *internal* organs but do not occur with breast radiation therapy.

Going through a combined course of surgery and radiotherapy is very demanding and should not be considered "easy" treatment. There must be rigid adherence to the radiation routine, 5 days a week for up to 6 weeks. A woman living in a smaller community without radiotherapy facilities may have to commute a long way each day, or even temporarily relocate. This is a big commitment of time and effort and requires emotional endurance. And first, there is the surgery. The cancerous tumor must be surgically removed. Enough tissue must be taken to remove the tumor and a small margin of surrounding tissue and for a hormone-receptor assay to be done. A separate incision must be made into the axilla so that lymph nodes may be examined and removed, if necessary. This is major surgery.

Removal of the lymph nodes (when having either a modified radical mastectomy or a lumpectomy) may cause certain aftereffects. Initially, there may be postoperative swelling and stiffness of the affected arm. This will decrease slowly until healing is completed. To keep swelling to a minimum, you should lie and sleep with your arm elevated for the next several weeks. Certain arm and finger exercises may be necessary to facilitate regaining full motion of that arm. In addition, extra care must be taken of the arm to avoid minor trauma which can cause swelling of the arm, even years later.

Doctors do not yet know if radiation therapy has any long-term harmful effects, especially for younger women. The evidence after 10 years does not indicate any later complications, but no figures are yet available for any effects 15 to 20 years later. Other parts of the body may be targets for x-rays, especially the thyroid, the colon, and the esophagus. There are no statistics to tell if these organs will or will not develop cancer at a later time because of the radiation. Such statistics can only be gathered after thousands of patients have been treated and then assessed over a longer period of time. Hopefully, with more accurate targeting of the radiation dose and with today's improved technology, changes in other organs will be minimal.

You and Your Treatment Alternatives

Today, when you are faced with the decision about treating local breast cancer, there is a range of choices available. Never before in the history of medicine have patients been so involved in choosing their treatments for something as serious as cancer. And never before have such crucial decisions been influenced by the emotionally charged issues of physical appearance, sexuality, and feminine identity. Most women will choose a treatment with a variety of intense feelings: anxiety about making so important a decision and about having a choice in something so vital in one's life; resentment at having to deal with a male physician when confronted with something so personal and frightening as the possibility of losing a breast; and confusion because of the array of treatment options.

In addition, at present, there is no single "right" or "best" way to treat local breast cancer. Physicians do not yet have the "final" answers, and this can be confusing and disturbing to many patients who for years have been accustomed to regarding their doctors as godlike authorities on health matters. Choosing the appropriate treatment for breast cancer has meant an enormous adjustment in how people relate to their physicians and in how physicians see themselves.

We think it is a very positive development that more and more weight is being given to the *quality* of a patient's life after she has been treated for breast cancer. This is, of course, bound to the issue of appearance, which for years was not given proper consideration. We have no doubt that the overwhelming significance of preserving the breast and all it entails physically and psychologically has become an enormous factor in women's choice of treatment. And that, in turn, has been instrumental in helping physicians become more attuned to their patients. Indeed, many doctors dealing with breast cancer have been gradually educated by their patients.

These emotional aspects of breast cancer treatment are crucial and should not be ignored. They should be discussed with your physician in an open way. If you are fearful about how you might feel if you were to lose a breast, you should bring this up. There are alternatives. If you would feel vulnerable and worried about removing a lump and having the remainder of your breast irradiated, you should discuss this with your doctor. You must consider your situation and *all* available options.

Some women, wanting more than anything else to "save" a breast, may opt for less extensive surgery. They may act because of unfounded fear or because they are misinformed, or they may make decisions based on emotions rather than on hard facts. This is a mistake.

In other words, emotional considerations alone should not be the *only* determinants of your treatment plan. Your treatment for breast cancer is far too important to be solely determined by a recent trend or fad or by unfounded fears and misconceptions. How well you will do with any treatment method depends on the specifics of *your* situation! Not all breast cancer patients are best served by *one* treatment method alone. You must have a complete evaluation of your own situation and should discuss your case with your physician and with other specialists if this helps you feel more knowledgable and comfortable. After your situation and the available options are thoroughly considered, the treatment plan best for *you* may be developed.

With any treatment plan there is a great deal of agreement about goals. All physicians agree that the primary aims in treating breast cancer are to preserve the woman's life, to minimize the chance of recurrence, and to provide the best cosmetic results possible. It is also generally agreed that the goal of disease control should not be compromised and should be the first priority.

However, there are differences of opinion concerning

treatment. Some physicians feel that not removing the entire breast may leave microscopic colonies of cancer cells in the remaining breast tissue. These microcolonies, if not eradicated, may eventually form additional tumors in the breast tissue left behind.

Other physicians, those favoring lumpectomy and radiation, feel that only a small percentage of microscopic cancer cells will ever become malignant tumor sites. They feel that radiation therapy following the lumpectomy will eradicate any microscopic disease that may remain behind after the primary tumor has been removed. If a recurrence does eventually occur, it can be treated by a modified radical mastectomy with good 5-year survival rates.

The lumpectomy-radiation treatment results have been studied for about 10 years. The survival rates are comparable to those of more extensive surgery. However, some doctors feel that cancer cells may recur as long as 15 to 20 years later. Therefore, longer trials are now being conducted.

How do you intelligently decide on a treatment plan that is best for you? How can you avoid making a decision based only on emotional factors and, instead, make a *rational* decision? It is essential to know as much as you can about your case. The only way you can do this is to obtain unbiased information from your doctor. For many women, this has been a difficult goal to reach.

About Physician Bias

Some women are concerned about physician bias when considering their options—concerned that they may get a different slant on their treatment choices depending on which physician they see when having a breast lump diagnosed. Such bias inevitably occurs when there are no conclusive answers, when various treatment approaches are valid, and where different specialists with different methods are involved in treating the disease. Most human beings, physicians included, will deal with a problem in a manner with which they are familiar and comfortable. Once established, the treatment method "takes hold," and only after long and arduous debate may new approaches gain acceptance. This is especially true when a patient's life hangs in the balance. In addition, today's super-specialization may occasionally foster tunnel vision in some specialists, narrowing their views of treatment alternatives.

Many patients feel, therefore, that they were not given adequate information about their treatment options. Indeed, some surgeons have steered their patients toward mastectomy without truly informing them of other available therapies. Some radiotherapists have minimized the uncertainties about local recurrence and the possible long-term effects of radiation when steering patients toward this option.

Because of such physician bias, some patients feel resentful, believing they were misled or that they "missed out," having undergone mastectomy without sufficient information about other choices. Others feel they were never given adequate information about reconstruction. The inescapable conclusion is that physicians often fail to help their patients learn about every available option. And sometimes, even when so informing their patients, these physicians make their bias undeniably evident. Although there is now more inter-specialty dialogue and cross-referring than before, a woman may encounter the problem of procedural bias when dealing with a lump in her own breast.

At present, five states—California, Hawaii, Massachusetts, Minnesota, and Wisconsin—have laws stating that breast cancer patients must be given complete information about *all* treatment alternatives. While medical objectivity cannot be legislated, such laws are ample evidence of the enormous impact physician bias about treatment methods has had on women and has influenced how they view their doctors.

How a patient can be assured of getting all the unbiased information she needs to make a treatment choice for her individual needs brings us to the issue of the *patient's role* and a *team approach* in understanding the viable options for treating breast cancer.

A Better Way

The choice of treatment for breast cancer ultimately rests with each patient. Any woman should be able to readily obtain a free flow of unbiased information provided in a straightforward manner. In our practices, we have developed a treatment team approach to accomplish this. If your surgeon works as part of a comprehensive treatment team, he or she has an available pool of specialists with whom you may consult regardless of the specific treatment you choose to have. This team includes a general surgeon, a radiotherapist, an oncologist, a plastic surgeon, and a psychiatrist.

In working as a group, these specialists recognize a patient's need for objective information when she is considering her treatment options. Though not all these specialists are necessarily needed by any one patient, they are available for consultation and have already established working relationships with each other. By sharing in the patient's diagnostic evaluation, they ensure that she learns all her treatment options and obtains the best possible care.

How can you best ensure that such a group approach is available to you? Since the first physician you will most likely be referred to is a surgeon, you must, at the outset, establish that you would like to examine *all* your treatment options before deciding which treatment you will have, if it becomes necessary. You should ask your surgeon for a referral to a radiotherapist with whom you can continue your fact-finding mission. By doing this you are already forming a potential treatment team even while considering your treatment choices.

If, after carefully considering your alternatives, you opt for one treatment plan over another, the same physicians may then proceed as a team with a good working relationship. You are not creating adversaries among the physicians who are explaining your treatment alternatives. You are engaging a team of doctors to advise and inform you of your choices so you can best proceed with your treatment. Keeping this team approach in mind will help you get the most expedient care with the least disruption in your life.

If at the outset you detect a bias in your surgeon's attitude or feel your doctor is not giving serious consideration to the various treatment alternatives, feel free to get a second opinion. Just within the last few years second opinions have become a standard and accepted part of medical practice. As a matter of fact, most insurance plans pay for a second opinion when you are considering treatment for any serious condition. Some patients, embarrassed to look elsewhere, feel they are somehow maligning the first doctor's professionalism or expertise by seeking another opinion. Others may feel a misguided sense of loyalty, thinking they are being "disloyal" to a doctor by looking elsewhere for information and possible treatment. This is not true. You are best off using the time between the biopsy and any proposed treatment to get all the information you can. Gathering information is vital; after all, the decision about treatment is ultimately yours.

We are well aware that the team approach is an ideal one not usually available to most women. Cross-referring and open-minded teamwork among various specialists who treat breast cancer is not yet the rule. It is rarely practiced by physicians unless patients ask for such referrals. Some patients find actively asking to be informed of their various options very difficult to do, especially when they do not have a long-standing relationship with the surgeon to whom they were referred. It may be helpful when first having a lump investigated by your family physician or gynecologist to inform *this* doctor of your wish to be referred to a surgeon who will open-mindedly consider *all* treatment options and who takes a team approach to the diagnosis and treatment of breast cancer.

Learning about Treatment; Making a Choice

When discussing the various treatment options with your team of physicians, you must make every effort to get as much information as you can. The following points are all relevant to making an intelligent treatment decision:

- The type of tumor you have
- The size of the tumor
- Its location on your breast
- The size and shape of your breast
- Your age and medical condition
- The treatment method you will feel most comfortable with when you consider both cosmetics and the long-term outlook

For instance, the type and size of tumor you have must be considered. How aggressive is it? How deeply infiltrated into the surrounding tissues is it? Is it very small so that it might be effectively removed by a lumpectomy?

The tumor's location within your breast is very important.
Is it in the upper, outer part? Near the nipple? Near the
breastbone? If it has developed in a location, such as behind
the nipple, where a lumpectomy will prove nearly as deform-
ing as a mastectomy, a lumpectomy may make very little
sense.

The size and shape of the tumor relative to the size and
shape of your breast must be taken into account. Is the
tumor large in comparison to the bulk of your breast, or
is it relatively small? If you have a small breast with a large
lump, a lumpectomy would involve removing a lot of breast
tissue. Your doctor then might recommend a mastectomy
since the lumpectomy itself would be tantamount to a mastectomy. Or your radiotherapist might feel that the tumor
is too large to radiate, so mastectomy might be best.

You must also consider your age and your medical condition. For instance, if you are in an older age bracket and
have a serious medical condition (other than the breast cancer) which could preclude your being a good candidate for
surgery, then the most minimal surgery possible would be
best.

There are other factors to be considered. For instance,
as we've said before, when being treated with radiation, there
is a certain amount of damage to normal tissue. No one
yet knows the long-term effects, if any, of this exposure on
the remaining breast tissue and on other organs. If, after a
lumpectomy with radiation, you eventually develop a recurrence of the tumor, you will then need a modified radical
mastectomy to eradicate the local disease.

Your emotional needs are also important. Will you feel
psychologically burdened by keeping part of a breast which
may again become cancerous in the future? If so, you might
not want anything less than total removal of the involved

breast. For you, mastectomy may be best, especially in view of the newer methods of reconstruction.

Or would you feel that less extensive surgery is less traumatic? If the issue of adjusting to breast loss is one you would rather avoid, then lumpectomy and radiation may be best for you.

Not every woman has *every* option, though the choices today are more varied than ever before. Sometimes your physical situation dictates what can or cannot be done in your case. Sometimes your psychological needs will prevail. Usually some combination of both will help you decide on your treatment.

Some women feel that having to decide is too great a burden and they may leave it to the doctor. Others feel that by having some say in the treatment plan, they are more in control of the situation, of their bodies, and of their lives.

The best treatment is the one you and your doctor agree is best for you!

Let's look at two patients we have treated to see how they decided on their treatment option.

❧ Pam Reimer described her choice:

"After the biopsy results came back, I was in a terrible state. My surgeon was really good. We had time to talk about what to do.

"I'd read all the articles about mastectomy—about how many breasts were cut off unnecessarily—and I'd never really thought much about it, at least not in relation to myself.

"After a while I began to see things differently. I wasn't so worried about losing the breast because I felt in a way that I had an ace up my sleeve—reconstruction. That was what helped me get through the whole thing.

"My surgeon told me about lumpectomy and radiation and he described the modified mastectomy. I think he was pretty neutral about which one I should choose, and I really think I had a choice. Two friends of mine had had mastectomies . . . one was nearly 10 years ago . . . and I think that influenced me. But when I really thought about it, I didn't want to take *any chance* at all. I couldn't bear the thought that I'd have a breast that could get cancer again, and I thought about radiation maybe giving me problems later on . . . in my 50s. You see, I'm a very *up* person. I was optimistic and I wanted to do what I thought would maximize my chances for the future. For me, it was a mastectomy and then . . . reconstruction."

🌹 Lucille Greene, who was 53 years old when the diagnosis of breast cancer was made, had a small tumor with no palpable lymph nodes in the axillary region on that side.

"I'd heard about women having a terrible time coping with mastectomy. I had to think of it in terms of my body and how I felt about it. And about myself. Even with breast reconstruction, it wouldn't really be *me*. I know my husband would love me no matter what, but I just felt that a mastectomy would have made me a different person in some way. I don't think I could have psychologically handled a mastectomy."

Lucille had a small, circumscribed lesion with fairly large breasts. It was not located near the nipple, so a lumpectomy could be done with good cosmetic results. There would be minimal deformity of the breast. The lumpectomy was performed along with an exploration of the regional lymph nodes in the axilla. Lucille's cancer was found to have spread to these nodes. She had Stage II cancer. At that point, her lymph nodes on the involved side were surgically removed.

"I was glad I chose the lumpectomy," Lucille said, reflecting back on her surgery, "because removing my breast probably wouldn't have made any difference. I learned that once it's in the lymph glands, there's a good chance it's already spread to the rest of the body and removing the breast is unnecessary. And if it hadn't gone beyond the nodes, then the x-rays could kill off the rest of the cancer."

Since Lucille had involvement of her axillary lymph nodes, she also had chemotherapy. She then went through a 6-week course of radiation treatment to the remaining breast tissue. Afterward, she received additional chemotherapy. It is now 3 years later, and she is doing very well.

"When I think back now at the age of 56, I'm thankful I didn't go for the mastectomy," said Lucille. "It would have been another hardship for me, and I think I'll do as well as I would have with a mastectomy. And I still have my breast."

Pam Reimer and Lucille Greene both had sufficient time to learn the facts of their situations and to explore their options. Then, in conjunction with their doctors, each realistically considered the physical and emotional issues and decided on a treatment plan.

Such active questioning and exploration is an entirely new role for many patients, but it is essential. Knowing which questions to ask (even before a problem develops), asking these questions, and asking for appropriate referrals can ensure that you learn about all possible options in your case.

Many women have told us that with all the emotional trauma of facing breast cancer, they were more able to deal with this crisis simply knowing they had a say in their treatment and that ultimately, there was a choice.

The Other Breast

Any patient treated for breast cancer may become concerned about her other breast. In many cases, breast cancer is a multifocal disease; it can occur in small microscopic areas throughout both breasts, either at once or over a period of years. Various studies of tissue from the opposite breasts of cancer patients have also revealed certain premalignant changes. Though these cells may never go on to develop into life-threatening tumors, the same factors are at work on the opposite breast as were working on the breast already treated for cancer.

The question remains about whether the opposite breast should be treated because it could potentially become cancerous.

Any patient treated for breast cancer should know that she is now at high risk for developing cancer in the other breast. The type of cancer treated in the first breast, the staging of the disease, the patient's age, and her family history of breast cancer are all important. So is the condition of the opposite breast. For instance, if that breast has multiple benign masses, it may be more prone to developing cancer. Also, such nodular breast tissue can make the detection of a new tumor difficult. Here, the mammography that was done to initially stage the breast cancer may serve as an excellent reference point for the follow-up of the opposite breast.

And there is the emotional state of the patient. She may have an excellent chance of cure because she discovered her tumor early, before there was any regional or bodywide spread. Yet she may live with the fear that this cure could be undone by an as-yet undetected new tumor in the opposite breast.

Still another concern is cosmetic. The treatment of the opposite breast depends to some extent on the kind of treatment given the diseased breast. If the patient has opted for radiation with minimal surgery, she may then be a candidate for radiation treatment of the opposite breast should it be necessary.

If the patient has had a mastectomy and contemplates reconstruction, sometimes the other breast may require treatment to allow for greater symmetry between the breasts. When the normal breast is much larger or if it sags, it may be altered to match the newly reconstructed breast.

When the patient is thought to be at high risk for developing cancer in the opposite breast, she may wish to consider having a subcutaneous mastectomy with cosmetic alteration of that breast. This operation removes the internal breast tissue, leaving the skin and nipple intact. A silicone gel implant is then inserted beneath the intact outer "shell" of the breast or beneath the underlying muscle. Cosmetic adjustments can be made for size, shape, and position of this breast so that it will be symmetrical to the reconstructed breast on the other side.

There is evidence that this operation can reduce the occurrence of cancer in the opposite breast, and for high-risk patients the statistical data about it is important. A large group of high-risk patients was studied. Although thought to be cancer-free, these patients had a 6 percent incidence of cancer when breast tissue was microscopically examined. There was also a 15 percent incidence of premalignant changes in the tissue. After subcutaneous mastectomy, the incidence of cancer dropped to about 0.5 percent. The statistics from this study are now under close scrutiny. Some physicians feel that 0.5 percent is too high a percentage of cancer occurrence to accept in a prophylactic operation. Other physicians feel that this operation, in addition to giving symmetry to the reconstructed breast, provides an additional measure of protection for the patient.

This operation cannot be recommended for every woman concerned about developing cancer in the opposite breast. But for the woman who is fearful because she is in the highest risk category (having had cancer in one breast and/ or having a strong family history of breast cancer), this procedure could alleviate much of her concern.

Some women who have never had breast cancer consult surgeons and request a subcutaneous mastectomy for prophylaxis against the possibility of developing the disease. These women usually have a very strong family history of breast cancer and, in addition, often have fibrocystic breast disease. Because of these increased risk factors, they may be good candidates for the procedure. Remember, a strong family history includes breast cancer occurring in two generations, with the cancer appearing in both breasts and developing before menopause. A history of one relative having unilateral breast cancer after menopause may not indicate a significantly higher risk than average.

To seriously consider prophylactic treatment, a woman should ask herself if her concern about developing breast cancer is so great that it is compromising her ability to lead a reasonably worry-free life. If this is so, then such a step may be reasonable. However, such a woman might also consider consulting a psychiatrist to make certain she is not focusing deeper emotional concerns in her life onto her breasts.

Prophylactic subcutaneous mastectomy is being done in selected cases by more and more surgeons. These physicians feel they are dealing with high-risk patients who may go on to develop life-threatening tumors. They take an aggressive surgical approach coupled with the idea of early recognition of the important high-risk factors. However, regardless of how thorough the surgeon may be in performing this procedure, some glandular tissue remains. There is a possibility that this tissue may someday develop cancer. The risks and benefits (this is major surgery with all its attendant risks) must be carefully examined before any procedure is planned.

In this chapter we have covered the basics about the various treatment options for your consideration. Your decision about treatment must be based on solid information about the details, benefits, risks, and limitations of each method, the specifics of your own case, and on any limitations your medical situation may impose. After you have learned all you possibly can about your condition, free of bias and misinformation, you may make a treatment choice based on your physical and emotional needs.

· *SEVEN* ·

Systemic Therapies
for Breast Cancer

Until a few years ago the responsibility for the management of breast cancer rested entirely in the hands of the surgeon. But breast cancer is not always a local disease strictly confined to the breast. In this chapter we will discuss *systemic* therapies, so called because they are used to combat and control cancer that has already gone beyond the breast to other systems or organs in the body.

Many physicians today are convinced that even when a tumor appears to be limited to the breast, some cancer cells may have already established themselves elsewhere in the body. These metastases may eventually multiply to form secondary growths in other organs. As mentioned in Chapter 6, when the regional lymph nodes are "positive" for cancer, it is more likely that cancer cells have spread to other parts of the body. However, these microcolonies of cancer cells do not always become secondary tumors.

No one knows why secondary tumors may develop in one patient but not in another. In the last few years, systemic treatments have been developed to treat these micrometastases in other parts of the body. Physicians feel that treating the entire "system" will improve the survival rates for women who have already been treated for an early, local breast cancer and whose lymph nodes are involved.

Two kinds of treatments are now used for systemic therapy: chemotherapy and endocrine therapy. Not all patients respond to either of these therapies, although about 60 percent of women respond to chemotherapy. Very often, it is the judicious use of combinations of chemotherapy and endocrine therapy that gives the best possible results.

These treatments may have serious side effects, and presently only women who most likely have metastases to other parts of the body are selected for systemic therapy. Therefore, chemotherapy and endocrine therapy are reserved for women who are "node positive" when their surgery is performed to control the local and regional disease. Someday, when effective chemotherapy with fewer serious side effects is available, all women diagnosed as having breast cancer may reasonably be candidates for this therapy.

Chemotherapy

Chemotherapy is treatment by drugs or chemicals that are cytotoxic (cell killers). Chemotherapy kills cancerous cells that have been shed into the body by the original breast cancer tumor or by a secondary tumor. The anticancer drugs circulate throughout the body, reaching cancer cells wherever they may have traveled.

But this therapy affects normal cells too, since no known anticancer drug exclusively attacks cancer cells. However, the important differences between cancer cells and normal cells—namely that the metabolic and growth patterns of cancer cells are much more rapid than those of normal cells—work to the healthy cells' advantage during chemotherapy. Anticancer drugs work during the duplicating period when the cancer cells' chromosomes are most vulnerable. Therefore, normal cells, which divide less frequently than cancer cells, are less susceptible to these drugs' effects.

Because all cancer cells within the body are not in the exact same stage of growth at the same time, drug therapy is given at various intervals to kill a maximum number of cancer cells. Chemotherapy is given orally or by injection into a vein. Treatments may be given weekly, monthly, and sometimes, on a daily basis. Most chemotherapy regimens today use various combinations of drugs to selectively kill cancer cells at a greater rate than normal cells are destroyed. But all anticancer drugs have potentially dangerous side effects and must be administered carefully by oncologists.

Side Effects

Normal cells in the body that have a higher turnover rate are most likely to be affected by these anticancer drugs along with the cancer cells themselves. Therefore, hair follicles, which grow rapidly, cells in the gastrointestinal tract, and the blood cells of the bone marrow are adversely affected during chemotherapy. Here are some of the major side effects of drugs used to combat cancer:

- Nausea and vomiting.
- Bone marrow depression. The bone marrow is the principal location for blood cell production. When the marrow is depressed, its ability to produce blood cells is inhibited and lowered. Generalized weakness and susceptibility

to infection may result. This reverses itself once the drug is stopped. At times during chemotherapy, the dose may have to be lowered if the blood count becomes too low.

- Hair loss (called *alopecia*). This is temporary. When the anticancer drugs are discontinued, the lost hair usually grows back, but it can be one of the most emotionally upsetting side effects of these medications.
- Interrupted menstruation.
- Irritability.

In addition, some patients who have these side effects for weeks or months may become emotionally depressed during chemotherapy treatment.

The side effects of these drugs are well known to oncologists now, and in most cases they can be anticipated and fairly well controlled.

Some Drawbacks

Anticancer drugs have varying degrees of toxicity and, in some cases, are even capable of causing leukemia in certain patients who have taken them for a long time.

Also, anticancer drugs may lose their cell-killing capacity as the body slowly builds up resistance to them. Delicate timing is needed to strike at the cancer cells when they are dividing, and constant monitoring by the oncologist is a must. This can be trying for the patient.

Despite these drawbacks, evidence now exists that in some patients, especially premenopausal women, these drugs are significantly improving survival time. They have been especially useful in cases where the cancer has already metastasized and formed secondary tumors. In the long run, oncologists hope to develop powerful chemotherapy agents that will have no side effects or complications—drugs that will selectively target and then destroy *only* cancer cells. At the present time, such medications are not available.

Endocrine Therapy

The endocrine glands are located at various internal areas of the body. They secrete hormones that are important for the regulation of many of the body's functions. In addition, certain hormones affect breast growth and function, and fairly often, the growth of breast cancer. Three such endocrine glands are the ovaries, the adrenal glands, and the pituitary gland.

Hormonal therapy, which manipulates the secretions of these glands, may be prescribed instead of or in addition to anticancer drugs for patients who develop secondary tumors that are influenced by hormones. At the time of the original biopsy, a hormone-receptor assay test is done to determine if the tumor depends on estrogen or progesterone for its growth. A tumor that depends on these hormones is termed *estrogen-dependent* or *progesterone-dependent*. If, at a later time, a secondary tumor develops, the levels of circulating hormones can be manipulated by antihormone medication. This deprives the new tumor of the hormone that helps it grow. About two-thirds of patients with estrogen-dependent tumors respond very well to endocrine therapy when a secondary tumor appears at a later time.

Until recently, surgical removal or radiation of the endocrine glands was used to decrease the level of circulating hormones and induce tumor regression once secondary lesions appeared. Today, surgery is no longer used for this purpose. Drugs known as antiestrogens are used to inhibit estrogen-dependent tumor growth. Tamoxifen™ is one of these drugs. So far, it has been used successfully in both pre- and postmenopausal women.

Combinations

Very often, a combination of treatments will most benefit a particular patient. The best combination requires a specific evaluation of a patient's tumor, its type, its degree of invasiveness, the extent to which it has spread, and its estrogen- or progesterone-dependent status, as well as a thorough evaluation of the patient by her physicians. Only then can an intelligent decision be made about which systemic treatment or combination of treatments will best work for that individual patient.

· *EIGHT* ·

Your Treatment: How to Deal with It

The Hospital

Any treatment you have for breast cancer will most likely require hospitalization. No matter how many times you have been to hospitals, being admitted for the treatment of breast cancer will very likely be a traumatic experience for you.

 "It happened so fast," said Barbara Conti. "There I was in the hospital and it was terribly real and frightening. I remember thinking, *This is it. I'm here because of breast cancer. It's really happening!* It was a terrible awakening because the reality of it hit me right there and then."

Most women feel perfectly well at the time of their admissions. This may add to the "strangeness" of entering a hospital. To feel healthy and be hospitalized for a serious disease seems a contradiction in terms.

Your reaction to being admitted to a hospital will no doubt depend on how you feel about hospitals, doctors, nurses, and illness in general. You may find it reassuring to think you are in the hands of trained and competent professionals. You may be concerned about the effect your hospital stay will have on child care, home care, money, job arrangements, and many other things. These can become especially important if you are single or divorced or if you contribute heavily to the family income. It is an even greater burden if you are the sole breadwinner in a household.

The change from normal routines upon the moment of admission can have an enormous impact. You may ordinarily be a resourceful wife, mother, homemaker, and career woman, and suddenly, you are thrust into the role of being a *patient*. You must take medication when directed; you must eat a restricted preoperative diet; visitors and activities will be limited.

In short, you must relinquish your everyday adult rights and privileges, and subordinate yourself to total strangers who are thoroughly familiar with this strange environment. You become dependent on the hospital and on the medical team in charge of your case. This is all a throwback to childhood, when your responsibilities were limited and so were your options. Naturally, different women will react differently to this situation, but whatever your normal life has been like, all this will require major emotional adjustments. Coupled with this is the ever-present knowledge of disease and of surgery. After all, hospitals are for sick people.

In our experience, one of the immediate concerns of patients about to undergo surgery is *anesthesia*. Fears range from worry about "losing control" to "dying while I'm under." Many patients openly express some fear that they may never awaken from their anesthesia. The time immediately preceding her mastectomy was very frightening for Pam Reimer.

"For 2 days before my surgery I had this nightmare about people dressed in white. I know it was the O.R. [the operating room] because they all had gowns and masks.

Everything was white, the gowns, the walls, the sheets . . . and I was lying there. And this mask was coming down over my face, like I was going to be smothered. And then, shaking all over, I'd wake up. It kept coming back to me— this dream—even after I was discharged. It took a few months to go away."

Communication is the key word. The hospital admission, the biopsy period, and the time before your surgery can be frightening and anguish-filled experiences. You must be willing to voice your concern to the members of your health care team. The more information you have about the various procedures, the less likely you are to feel ignored, anxiety-ridden, and pessimistic.

In our view, your emotional needs at this time are just as important as your medical requirements. Being hospitalized is an emotional experience as much as it is a physical or medical one. Many women are reluctant to discuss their worries with a surgeon or a nurse. They may fear they will be viewed as silly or self-indulgent for taking up valuable time with nonmedical questions or complaints. They may believe that stoic silence is the only thing a patient should display in a hospital. Nothing could be more wrong! Most patients who have terrible hospital experiences find various *nonmedical* aspects of the situation the most distressing of all.

For instance, there is a very impersonal quality to being a patient on a busy ward. You may be one of many people admitted that day. Your presence is not terribly significant to many of the people around you. The maintenance worker who cleans the floor is not going to be especially tuned in to your needs or fears. The technician who draws your blood each morning may not be the model of sensitivity and compassion. The dietary aide handing you your meal tray will probably not be concerned about your emotional well-being. We aren't saying that these people will be unpleasant, but they will probably not take much personal interest in you no matter how difficult a time this is for you.

This impersonal quality may be the perfect soil in which your fears and worries may flourish. Don't let silence and lack of information make your fears expand.

Certain common worries emerge with nearly every breast cancer patient. You may worry about how the operation will proceed. You may wonder how a mastectomy will affect your looks, your well-being, and your relationship with your husband. How will it affect your relationship with your friends, your sexual life, your activities, the clothing you wear, and your entire view of yourself? How will having cancer affect your sense of the future? All these and other concerns may surface as soon as you are admitted to the hospital.

Even if you're the strong, silent type, you may suddenly find yourself "letting go" with more feelings than you ever thought you had stored up inside yourself. If you *do* show your feelings—anger, fear, sadness, and others—accept them for what they are. They are a part of you at this time. Don't be upset because they have surfaced. Your situation is probably more difficult and demanding than any other you have ever faced.

You will react in your own way to this physical and emotional life crisis. How you cope will partly depend on how you have coped with past problems in your life. If you've never felt free to discuss your feelings, it will be difficult for you to do so at this time. If you've always freely brought out your feelings, you have an advantage here.

You must know what to expect before your operation. You should talk with your anesthesiologist to learn whatever you need to know about anesthesia. Nowadays, a sedative is often given while patients are still in their rooms, which induces a pleasant state of drowsiness and alleviates anxiety.

You should speak with your surgeon to learn all you need to know about your operation. No doubt, these issues will already have been discussed in your consultation with your surgeon, but reinforcement of the information at this time can be very helpful. Many surgeons and hospitals employ nurse-oncologists who can provide additional help. They are aware of the overall course of your treatment, and their role as liaison between the busy ward activities and your own personal care can be very comforting.

Having talked with your surgeon means you should, at this point, know the answers to the following questions about your surgery: What will the operation entail? How long will it take? What can I expect once I get out of the recovery room? What side effects or partial incapacitation might I experience after having a mastectomy? Will I have pain? How long will this take to resolve? What possible complications are involved? What will my postoperative course be like?

Knowing what to expect can be especially helpful if you are going to have a mastectomy. Some patients find it helpful if, during their preoperative consultations, they are shown photographs of other patients who have had mastectomies, giving an approximation of how they will look after surgery. This helps because rarely is the actual postoperative look as terribly disfiguring as you may imagine beforehand it will be.

At this time it is usually a good idea to have at least one family member present for emotional support. You may be anxious and upset during all the preoperative preparations, and having your husband or another relative close by can prevent your forgetting or distorting the important details of your preoperative consultation. Remember, breast cancer is a family crisis. Those close to you will very much want and need to be with you.

Dealing with surgery requires emotional strength and a willingness to confront unpleasant and sometimes frightening realities. Remember, *the desire to fight cancer is vital to your outcome.* It is every bit as important as your treatment itself.

Adjusting to Mastectomy

Having a mastectomy requires making adjustments, both psychological and physical, before and after surgery.

Once you are out of the recovery room and back in your hospital room, your physical and emotional recovery must begin. Over a short period of time you will regain your strength and your surgical wound will heal. The area affected by surgery is usually covered with a dressing. There may be drains to collect fluid from the operative site. Remember, *any* surgery or intervention into the body's tissues will result in some swelling and discomfort. It will take time for this to subside and for the wound to heal.

It is not unusual for physical sensations to be present in the area where the breast was removed. There may be tingling, pins-and-needles sensations, and discomfort. These sensations usually disappear gradually, and you will regain your presurgical level of activity with no discomfort.

Perhaps the most important part of your postoperative period is coping with the emotional issues associated with losing a breast and having a serious disease.

For some patients, the time right after surgery is very difficult. Having lost a breast now assumes a degree of reality it never had before. Some patients suddenly become aware of their own mortality and of the possibility of death. Others may want to avoid (by denying) these unpleasant associations. They may drop the word *cancer* from their vocabularies or refuse to discuss their conditions. Sometimes this is helpful, for a while—if it is not carried to an extreme.

Anxious concerns about your future and well-being may now surface again. These anxieties are normal and the incision scar may very well be a reminder of all these issues. Many women have described being reluctant or frightened to look at their incision scars soon after a mastectomy. The time for the first dressing change can be very trying. Again, it will be helpful if you have already seen photographs of mastectomy scars; you won't feel shocked, and your expectations will not be influenced by your imagination. (See photograph on page 127.) Some women say it helps to take gradual looks each time the dressing is changed over the course of the first few postoperative days. Remember that the scar will look better as time passes and the incision wound heals. Recall too how Pam Reimer felt she had an "ace up her sleeve" because she knew she had the option of breast reconstruction at a later time. Some patients arrange to have reconstructive surgery done along with their mastectomies. We will discuss this in Chapter 10.

Some women react to their mastectomies with anger and resentment. Some anger is probably normal and quite healthy, and if you can ventilate it, you can deal with it much more effectively than if it smoulders deep inside you. Bottled-up, seething feelings will only surface later, at a time when they may be more intense and possibly more damaging. Letting out some angry feelings may actually help you turn your thoughts toward recovery and rehabilitation. In our view, anger is less intense and less damaging if you

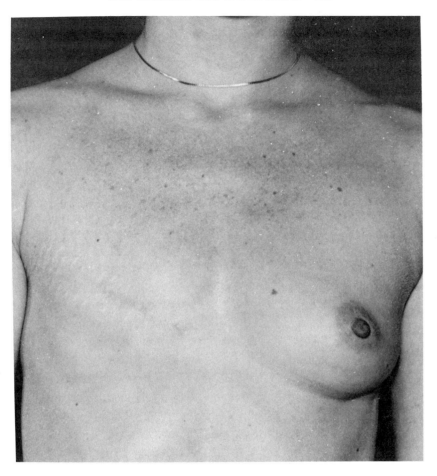

*This 40-year-old woman had a modified radical mastec-
tomy of the right breast. Her mastectomy scar shows
cross-hatching. Today, it is possible to have results with
less prominent scarring because general surgeons often
confer with plastic surgeons in an effort to minimize
scar formation.*

have been prepared for your surgery and if you have known the facts and options of your case.

When you lose a breast, your body image, the way you see yourself, is altered, and this requires getting used to. The extent to which you may feel "devalued" or "damaged" will partly depend on how much value you place on your breasts as a measure of self-esteem and sexual desirability. It is well known that a woman whose self-worth is based on her physical appearance is more likely to be depressed after mastectomy than a woman whose self-esteem is derived from other attributes such as professional achievement or family.

Here, too, many women find it helpful to think beyond the scar and the missing breast. They may already think about a breast prosthesis and about breast reconstruction. In our opinion, the possibility of breast reconstruction has significantly changed the emotional equation for women who have lost a breast. Today, many patients choose to consult with a reconstructive surgeon *before* a mastectomy. Asking your general surgeon for a referral to a reconstructive surgeon means using the team approach, which can make the entire process less ominous and help you make a better adjustment to mastectomy. For some women, positive thoughts about having a breast reconstructed may be the first glimmerings of restoring and reconstructing themselves psychologically.

For Pam Reimer breast reconstruction was a "given," even before she had her mastectomy.

❧ "There was no way I wasn't going to have reconstruction," Pam said more than a year after her mastectomy. "I wanted to have it along with the surgery, or right afterwards, but my surgeon wanted me to wait until everything healed. I know that thinking about it [reconstruction] helped me get through the whole thing. It was the most important thing to me . . . it helped me cope."

Pam Reimer always placed great value on her looks. For her, it was unimaginable to go through life with only one breast, and her focusing on reconstruction even before mastectomy was a healthy and adaptive response to an intolerable (for her) disfigurement.

It is not unusual to become depressed following a mastectomy. Depression will vary depending on your age, your life situation, your ability to deal with stress and loss, and on your relationships with your family and your surgeon. There can be little doubt that if you have a loving partner and a rich family life and if you've been informed and prepared for surgery, you will be less likely to feel depressed than if you live alone and have had poor communication with your doctor and other members of your medical team.

Some depressive feelings are normal. To anyone, the loss of a body part is equivalent to losing someone or something that is valued or loved. Grieving is an appropriate reaction when you have lost someone you love, or when a breast has been removed. Only if grieving escalates and turns into self-loathing thoughts and feelings is it serious enough to warrant consultation with a psychiatrist.

Some women may not be depressed after the operation, and several months later are surprised when they see an evening gown with a low-cut neckline and they feel saddened. Usually this depressive feeling is brief and not too intense.

Some breast cancer patients may appear cheerful and even elated immediately after surgery. This may be the first important postoperative sign that a patient is not responding appropriately to a real-life loss and to real danger in the form of a serious disease. Overactivity, excessive talkativeness, and elation may mean the patient is having a postoperative "high." This can be a sign of masked depression or even of mania, and a psychiatrist should be available in any such situation.

The important signs and symptoms of depression are:

- Lowered self-esteem—feelings of worthlessness, guilt, hopelessness, and helplessness.
- Feelings of fatigue; lack of energy; appetite disturbances, often accompanied by weight loss or gain, and sleep disturbances—usually waking up very early and not being able to get back to sleep.
- Turning inward; concentrating on vague bodily sensations and symptoms, becoming fearful of disease, restricting one's activities and constantly worrying about one's health. This is hypochondria.

In summary, after a mastectomy, you may very likely have a variety of unpleasant thoughts and feelings. This is *normal.* You may feel anxious about the future and about your health. You may be fearful about the chance of a recurrence. You may feel angry, as though you were "singled out" for all this. You may feel that your body has been disfigured and that you'll never look as good as you once did. You may feel worry, loss, grief, and depression about your disease and about what has happened to you. These feelings and thoughts are *all* normal. They are normal so long as they don't become extreme or too intense and providing they don't dominate the way you think, feel, and interact with other people.

It is a mistake to think that you should accept the loss of your breast as a matter-of-fact occurrence. You will go through a difficult period of adjustment. This will vary from one woman to another depending on many factors. As we've said, one of the most important determinants in this adjustment period is your family. The support and understanding of the people who love you can go a long way toward your emotional adjustment and a positive view toward your future.

Within any well-thought-out treatment team for breast cancer patients, a psychiatrist should be available for consultation if the patient requests it. In our experience, when patients are made aware that psychological counseling is available even *before* it may be needed, they feel reassured by this extra measure of emotional support. While many patients adjust to the stressful circumstances of the hospital and surgery, some may feel the need to talk with a trained professional.

A Group Approach

Going through a mastectomy causes many women to reevaluate their life-styles and goals. Many self-help groups have formed in recent years, which attempt to bring women together to discuss their feelings about breast cancer, about mastectomy, and about the emotional concerns they may have following this course of treatment. These groups have helped many women feel better about themselves by knowing that hundreds of thousands of women have gone through the same experience and are doing very well.

The American Cancer Society's Reach to Recovery program is among the better known group support systems. In many hospitals, with your physician's consent, you may be visited soon after your mastectomy by a volunteer from Reach to Recovery. This woman will be supportive and understanding, and she will provide you with literature and advice about exercises, prostheses, clothing, and many other aspects of rehabilitation. The most notable thing about Reach to Recovery volunteers is that they themselves have had a mastectomy for breast cancer.

Such supportive help from women who are sympathetic and familiar with your feelings and thoughts can be very helpful. The mere presence of a volunteer in your hospital room soon after your surgery may be reassurance that you are not alone. And even more important, you can know from talking with your volunteer that rehabilitation is possible. Reach to Recovery also provides your husband and other family members with a letter that attempts to help them understand some of what you may be experiencing at this time.

In addition to the trained ACS Reach to Recovery volunteer, an increasing number of hospitals now have postmastectomy rehabilitation groups. Some programs provide self-help groups along with individual counseling sessions for patients, their partners, and other family members to help them all cope with anxieties about breast cancer. Other programs provide registered nurses who visit patients after surgery to teach BSE and discuss various types of breast prostheses.

Many rehabilitation programs are available for women and their husbands. Some mastectomy rehabilitation groups are offered by organizations such as local "Y"s and by various state divisions of the American Cancer Society. There are counseling groups all over the country, often formed by people (women *and* men) who have felt their emotional needs were not fully met by more organized societies. Also some surgeons, in conjunction with a psychiatrist, have organized group discussions for their own patients.

To get information about the availability and location of these groups and organizations, you can telephone the National Cancer Institute in Bethesda, Maryland. The telephone service is staffed by trained supervisors and volunteers who have extensive, up-to-date information about every aspect of cancer, including rehabilitation, and will provide you with information about resources and services in your area, anywhere in the United States. To use this service call or write:

Cancer Information Clearinghouse
Office of Cancer Communications, National Cancer Institute
7910 Woodmont Avenue, Suite 1320
Bethesda, Maryland 20014
(301) 496-4070

Coping with Radiation Therapy

The emotional aftereffects of surgery may be compounded if you need additional treatment after leaving the hospital. Radiation treatments mean interrupting your return to a normal home environment. You may have to return to the treatment facility nearly every day for 5 or 6 weeks. Fortunately, most patients receiving radiation therapy have had surgical lumpectomy, which may be less physically and psychologically traumatic than a mastectomy.

You should not misinterpret your radiation therapy as a sign that "something else is wrong with me" or that "my condition has worsened." In most cases, radiation treatment is a preplanned part of your treatment protocol, although for some patients, this follow-up radiation may be decided on after surgery has been done.

❧ Pam Reimer found herself in this situation. Although her axillary lymph nodes were not lumpy on her presurgical examinations, at surgery an incision was made into her axilla on the side of the breast cancer. Cancer cells were found in several lymph nodes. Even though these nodes were barely involved, the disease was not regarded as Stage II breast cancer. Pam's surgeon and the radiologist agreed it would be advisable for her to have radiation to the rest of her nodes after her mastectomy.

This was a frightening surprise to Pam, who had, until then, thought her cancer was confined to her breast. Her anxiety escalated and soon was as intense as when the diagnosis was first made.

Pam's husband told us that during her radiation treatments, she became more depressed than during any other phase of this ordeal. She became very pessimistic, feeling the need for radiation was an indication that she had "advanced" cancer with widespread involvement of the rest of her body. Fortunately, much of this subsided after Pam finished her treatment.

Many patients are fearful of radiation therapy. Some fear they will be "burned." Others fear they will be made "radioactive" and will then be contaminated or that other people will be concerned about this and will avoid them. These worries are myths, which are best dispelled before radiation therapy is begun.

There is no doubt that radiation therapy itself can cause anxiety. The machine is ominous-looking, and you are sealed off in a room away from other people. The best way to avoid anxiety is to have your physician fully explain the treatment procedure *before* you have your first treatment session. Your family should be included in these talks. Then, they will be less likely to form ideas based on misconceptions about radioactivity or "contamination." You should know how radiation works against cancer and which side effects you may develop. Then, if during your treatments you experience mild nausea, a lump in your throat, fatigue, or skin changes in the irradiated area, you will know that the radiation is causing these effects, not a recurrence of the cancer.

Knowing how to deal with certain problems that may arise is essential. You may have nausea and vomiting once in a while. Small, frequent meals may help counteract this. So will fruit punch, carbonated beverages, and soups. You must maintain a good caloric intake and do the best you can to eat nutritious meals for the 5 or 6 weeks during radiotherapy.

During treatment you should avoid exposing the treated area to the sun. Check with your physician before applying any ointments or soaps.

Coping with Chemotherapy

Chemotherapy has been used for some time to treat breast cancer in its more advanced stages and some physicians are now beginning to use it as an adjunct to surgery for the treatment of primary or even early breast cancer. This is not a widespread practice, but there may be a time when new anticancer drugs are found which have few or no side effects. If this happens, we can expect to see more breast cancer patients receiving chemotherapy as a routine part of the treatment for early breast cancer.

Some patients become pessimistic when they learn they are candidates for chemotherapy. As we mentioned earlier, this treatment is usually given to patients whose cancer involves the axillary lymph nodes in addition to the breast. It is also given when cancer is more advanced and has spread to other parts of the body. Chemotherapy is used to destroy any metastasized cells and prevent their possibly developing into secondary tumors. It is important to realize that even if cancer cells are deposited throughout the body, they may not form secondary tumors, even without chemotherapy. Actually, many patients view their chemotherapy as a kind of "mopping up" to make sure all cancerous cells are killed.

The various side effects often associated with chemotherapy, along with visits to the hospital for the treatments, can delay any semblance of life returning to normal. Before beginning chemotherapy you should discuss your treatment with your oncologist. You should know about the benefits, risks, and side effects of chemotherapy and how they will affect your life. Close family members should be included in these discussions so they will know what you may be going through. This will lesson the possibility of misunderstanding between you and your family if side effects interfere with your ability to function normally.

If during your chemotherapy you have nausea and vomiting, small, frequent meals will help. So will carbonated beverages. Avoid overly sweet or rich foods; they can make things worse. So will eating too quickly or overexertion.

You may experience temporary loss of, or changes in, taste and smell sensations, which may make it more difficult to want to eat, especially if there is nausea. In addition, you may occasionally develop sores in your mouth.

Some chemotherapy regimes cause diarrhea. You must avoid foods such as bran, whole cereals, and vegetables with roughage. You should drink lots of fluids since you will need to replace potassium lost because of diarrhea.

Most of all, you may have to bear up under the emotional burden of feeling unwell during various parts of your chemotherapy.

🌺 Lucille Greene, who had a lumpectomy along with radiation and chemotherapy, talked about her chemotherapy three years later.

"It was the worst part. It was certainly the longest and most involved. And the side effects were terrible. I always felt sick, weak, and tired. It affected my whole life. I couldn't keep up with the housework. I had no enthusiasm for anything . . . for television, for my family . . . for anything. For a while I questioned if it was worth it—if anything could be worth what I was going through. I got very depressed, especially when my hair fell out. I hated that wig. I thought it was the ugliest thing I ever saw. I think it symbolized the whole treatment and how everything in my life was wrong.

"We went through a lot together, my husband and me. And in certain ways we're better off for it—at least *now* I think so. That's part of what's so strange about all this. After you've gone through it, you forget the pain and the turmoil. Most of it. I guess when I look back now, it turned out all right. I never thought I'd hear myself say this, but I think I was lucky. It could have been worse."

The Need for Follow-Up

Part of dealing with breast cancer is recognizing and accepting the need for medical follow-up. It is equally important to practice monthly self-examination.

Your visits to your doctor may be an unpleasant reminder of the possibility of the cancer recurring; it is certainly part of a process of acknowledging the disease and its impact on your life. Your actual schedule of visits must be individualized. Many doctors prefer having visits set at every 3 months during the first 2 years, every 6 months for the next 3 years, and at 1-year intervals after that.

Each visit should involve a thorough physical examination. The area of the incision scar and the other breast must be carefully examined along with the axillary lymph nodes. You should also have annual laboratory tests, including blood count, urinalysis, chest x-rays, and so on. Your doctor may want you to have a mammogram of your remaining breast each year.

Once you have been diagnosed as having breast cancer, you must be vigilant and pursue an ongoing course of medical follow-up for the rest of your life.

· NINE ·

How Has My Life Changed?

❧

No matter what treatment you have had for breast cancer, you will most likely return to a family setting. Returning home can be very trying, and nearly every woman who has had this disease knows it deeply affects those close to her. The problems don't end with your discharge from the hospital. For some women, difficulties seem to begin on the day they return home. In this chapter we will explore the difficulties and concerns our patients most often encounter, ones which often lead them to ask certain questions about their relationships with people and about how things have (and have not) changed.

You and Your Family

The people in your family may also suffer through an ordeal during the time your cancer was diagnosed and then treated. Shock, denial, and anger at the diagnosis may be the most easily noticed. Along with these feelings may be others that are less obvious because people don't necessarily talk about them or even admit them to themselves. Your husband and children may feel guilt-ridden about your situation, even wondering if they "contributed" to your illness. They may feel remorse for having missed opportunities to tell you how they really feel about you. Sometimes these feelings can complicate relationships because they are partly based on the assumption that you are gravely ill and may die.

As a matter of fact, ignorance about cancer is often the cause of most fears expressed by cancer patients and their families. Many people assume that cancer is always fatal, and this may lead to guilty feelings. You may actually have an optimistic personal outlook and prognosis about your treatment and rehabilitation, and yet, your family may be thinking, feeling, and acting as though you were dead or about to die! Beware of this and beware the family setting where silence prevails, where nothing is *really* discussed and where apprehension or unnecessary pessimism grows.

Just as in the detection and treatment phases of this experience, not-knowing and poor communication are your (and your family's) enemies. By not talking about your disease you are *not* protecting your family. You are not sparing them anything unpleasant. Instead, you may be doing just the opposite. Not communicating means allowing a pattern of mutual deception to develop. This may also be called a conspiracy of silence. Silence and deception will only foster vagueness, ignorance, and eventually, mistrust.

They aren't being real with me, is how some patients begin to feel. *They lie to me,* is another feeling. *They pretend it's all right, that nothing is wrong, but I'm worried,* is how someone else may express it. If this kind of silence and denial take over, talking about your concerns becomes much more difficult, and then, more silence prevails.

Your family must understand that you cannot silently cope

with your burden alone. You will suffer the most if you actually want to talk about your disease and your feelings but do not—or feel you cannot—because you are trying to protect your family's feelings. You may feel forced into the role of bolstering everyone else's morale when *you* may be the one needing the comfort and support at this time. If you do not get this support, you and your family may unintentionally abandon each other emotionally. You will feel rejected.

Sharing thoughts and feelings about your illness must be given priority at this time. A family that refuses to face your diagnosis of breast cancer, one that cannot acknowledge your fears and its own or has trouble accepting them, one that doesn't give you the love and support you now need will seriously hinder your ability to cope with your situation.

Family members and friends of cancer patients often fear they don't know what to say to the patient. Honest thoughts and feelings should be expressed. This may sometimes be difficult, and if it is, there are other ways of expressing feelings. A held hand, a look, a touch, or a gesture is sometimes much more expressive than any conversation can be.

Patients' Concerns

In the remainder of this chapter we will discuss the issues our patients bring up most often. These worries and concerns are frequently expressed as anxious questions.

Will I always live with the fear of recurrence? Can I make long-range plans?

There is no question that, in some ways, your life has changed. You have had a brush with your own mortality, and you will never forget it. We cannot say you will never

have a recurrence of cancer; that would be an absurd prediction. Some women die of breast cancer. Your prognosis
depends on the many factors we discussed earlier, but you
need not live in *fear* of recurrence. Naturally, some anxiety
and fear are perfectly appropriate at first. Many women report that fear was greatest just after they discovered their
lump. Others report they were very fearful and depressed
right after their surgery.

As time passes, you will adjust to living with the idea of
breast cancer and its implications. Your anxiety and fear
will subside providing you have a supportive and positive
family setting after your treatment. Naturally, if you are receiving chemotherapy or radiation, your return to a more
normal environment and feelings will be prolonged.

❦ Fear of recurrence is quite common, and most women
have reactions similar to Pam Reimer's during the first year
of her recovery.

"I was worried all the time . . . about every little thing.
A cough, a cold, the slightest pain, especially if it was in
the chest. There was one time when I coughed very hard
and up came a small amount of blood. I panicked.
Completely. Even after my doctor explained that a small
capillary probably broke from the coughing, it didn't reassure
me. He told me I was all right and after about a week, I
calmed down.

"Now, it's a year later and I'm not as tuned into my body
as I was then. I hardly even think about it now. As a matter
of fact, I just got over a cold and it didn't even worry me.

"But the way I felt last year at this time . . . if anyone
had ever told me that I'd be going about my life normally,
that I wouldn't be worried about getting sick and dying,

I'd have thought they were crazy. At that time, I was really a hypochondriac. You know . . . after a while you make the adjustment."

❦ Barbara Conti put it differently.
"I can't say it was easy, but after 12 years, I've got a perspective that I didn't have at first. For the first year I thought I'd never be able to cope. I was depressed, worried, pessimistic . . . you name it. No matter what I was involved with, I saw everything as though I was looking down a long tunnel . . . and the tunnel was called cancer. Or maybe it was called mastectomy. That dominated my thinking. But I've come a long way now, and I'm cured."

Most physicians feel that if you have been symptom-free for 5 to 10 years after your treatment with no evidence of recurrence, your chances of a normal life span are excellent. In many physicians' experiences, the patients who fare best when being treated for cancer of any kind seem to be those who make long-range plans and who strive for certain goals. A recent film, *Champions,* is the true story of an English steeplechase jockey who at the beginning of the film discovers he has cancer. He suffers through a long and difficult treatment of surgery and chemotherapy, planning all the while to return to the horse-racing circuit. He has a woman who loves him, a sister who cares, and an employer who is understanding. Through it all, he is convinced he will eventually return and win the Grand National. His rousing story is a testament to his determination and his will to fight, and win.

A book called *We the Victors* tells the true stories of patients who fought cancer and won. A particular quality seems common to them all. Each in his or her way had formed a long-range goal or plan of some kind. Each strived for something important in the future. One patient wanted to live long enough to see a young sapling she had planted grow into a tree large enough to shade her house. Another, a former basketball player who had lost a leg to bone cancer, made plans to eventually play basketball again. And he did!

Each of these people had a concrete goal; each had something to strive for. Perhaps such goal setting was the natural result of an unquenchable desire to live and succeed. And perhaps such desire triggers some as-yet-unknown mechanisms of immunity or resistance to disease. No one really knows. We aren't saying that the will to live and striving for goals will guarantee victory over cancer; advanced cancer very often has a poor prognosis. But people with a will to fight and live for a meaningful future often survive cancer and live fruitful lives.

Barbara Conti had been a school teacher for many years when she developed cancer. She had a supportive husband, who helped her get through her treatment and its emotional aftermath. (Recall her experience at Bloomingdale's.) Two years after her surgery she decided to become an assistant principal. Over the next few years she took courses, passed examinations, and eventually did become an assistant principal. Now, 12 years after her initial diagnosis, she still looks to the future and a possible position as the principal of a grade school in her community.

Pam Reimer continued working as before. In addition, she became very involved with the Reach to Recovery program after her own treatment for breast cancer.

Lucille Greene became active in her local "Y," where she helped form a program in group counseling for cancer patients and their families. She also decided she wanted to pursue other interests and is now completing a course for licensure as a real estate broker. "I think my illness was the springboard I needed," said Lucille. "It put me into gear and gave me the courage to strive for something I'd always wanted to do."

What about depression? Is it normal? How do I cope with it? Will it go on for a long time?

Depression, grief, and sadness are all normal reactions to a severe loss. Breast cancer means dealing with the possibility of losing your life and with the loss of a breast—if you have a mastectomy without reconstruction. If you are somewhat younger, this brush with mortality and the realization that your health is compromised (though not lost) can be very depressing.

Many patients are depressed after surgery; the reality of the situation may hit home then. Others find that depression sneaks up on them later, when they have been home for a while. A dominant feeling is, *My whole life has changed for the worse and there's nothing I can do about it.* There can be overwhelming feelings of helplessness and hopelessness.

❦ For some months after returning home from the hospital, Pam Reimer had periods of intense depression. These were discrete periods of sadness, crying, and feelings of despair—they weren't constant. Pam still worked at the law firm and was very much a wife and mother.

"I would sometimes spend hours and hours looking in the mirror at my scar, and believe me, I had plenty of good cries over it," said Pam. "There were times, not all the time, just moments or minutes, sometimes longer, when I didn't know how I'd get through the day. When I couldn't believe I'd ever make it or that I'd ever feel right again."

Having cancer, losing a breast, acknowledging you have such an illness may reactivate depressing feelings from past times: for example, sorrow over the loss of a parent or the death of someone you cared about from long ago. Some other meaningful loss may suddenly surface in feelings, even though your bad feelings at the moment are connected only with your breast cancer. Or breast cancer and the feelings it evokes may color the present so that even a minor loss or disappointment may take on an intensity it otherwise wouldn't have.

Most women say their depressed feelings come and go, that they aren't by any means constant. There may be moments when they well up—while shopping in a store; watching television, a play, or a film; hearing an old song—but the feelings usually fade.

You must expect to have occasional difficulties during this adjustment to a new reality in your life. Part of your emotional task at this time is to make peace with the idea of your own mortality. Also, for the next 5 to 10 years you must accept the possibility of your cancer recurring. And you must find new resources within yourself so you can feel worthy of being loved and fulfilled in your life. These aren't easy tasks, especially when depression is part of the picture.

There can be added difficulty if breast cancer strikes at the time you are going through menopause. The physical effects of menopause may themselves compound the problem. The time when a woman ceases to have her periods can be difficult, since menstruation is associated in people's minds with the idea of femininity, motherhood, and ability to bear children. Menopause is a natural milestone in life, one which for some women can be difficult, especially if children have grown up and are moving away. A woman who has had few other areas of activity or sources of self-esteem may get depressed. Still, most women cope with this life milestone and find new ways to define themselves.

Naturally, accomplishing this while coping with cancer and depressed feelings is easier if you have the support of a loving and caring family. In addition, the understanding of relatives, friends, coworkers, and your doctor can all be very helpful. We have found that many breast cancer patients have friends who themselves have been treated for breast cancer. There is, of course, a meaningful commonality among women who have had the same disease. Such friends can provide helpful support.

If depression becomes too insistent or intense, you must get proper counseling and treatment. A group setting, available through your local "Y" or through local chapters of various cancer organizations, can be helpful, but occasionally, some people may need counseling or antidepressant medication administered by a psychiatrist. If your surgeon has been working as part of a comprehensive treatment team, you may already have met with a psychiatrist or been advised of this physician's availability. In any event, your surgeon should be able to provide you with the name of a psychiatrist who is familiar with the kinds of feelings breast cancer and mastectomy evoke in most women. Such a referral—if you ask for it—may be vital to your success in dealing with your treatment. As we've said before, depression itself is not abnormal in these circumstances. Only if it becomes too intense or prolonged and interferes with your life does it require medical treatment.

If you are a single or divorced woman dealing with the physical and emotional concerns of breast cancer, your task may be more difficult. Certainly, living alone and not having a caring partner make coping and readjusting harder. But there are still relatives and friends. You may make use of the various group and individual counseling resources in your community. And there is yourself; you must find inner resources you perhaps never before knew you possessed. For you, the setting of new personal and professional goals may be crucial to your well-being and to your having the sense of a meaningful future.

What about my relationship with my husband? How about sex? Will he be turned off? Interested in other women? Will he feel obligated to me out of pity? What will become of us?

Your partner will play an important part in your experience with breast cancer. A husband's reaction, or the anticipation of his reaction, to the issues of cancer and breast loss is often critical to a woman's emotional well-being, for it affects her own feelings about that loss. Most women will interpret a negative response as a kind of rejection. Avoidance may be interpreted as pity. If a partner is supportive and caring, a woman's reaction to all this may be helped enormously.

If you have had a mastectomy, there is no doubt that your partner will respond to it. In our experience, most husbands respond much more positively than their wives expect. A favorable response doesn't mean your husband will have *no* response. It is perfectly normal for a partner to have a variety of complicated feelings when he first looks at the operative scar. There may be shock, disappointment, and sorrow. These are normal feelings.

Most husbands are concerned about how they may react

to the wound and wonder what response is appropriate. Some men will be curious. Some deliberately avoid looking at it. Some women try to avoid the issue completely. For nearly a year, Pam Reimer covered her scar in the presence of her husband.

🌹 "I bought lots of sexy night clothes," Pam said. "But every one of them had a matching top. I didn't want my husband to see me that way . . . I don't know why. I guess *I* couldn't stand seeing myself with one breast, and I didn't want him to see it either. He didn't ask to see it; maybe that was my clue. He told me over and over that he didn't care about the breast, that it wasn't important to him. He joked and said he was a 'tush man' anyway, that he didn't care about the breast, that all he cared about was that I was alive.

"I guess I believed him, but it took a while. I had to be convinced. When I got home from the hospital I was very uptight about making love. I know I expected him to reject me, and I was unsure about everything. We didn't do anything for nearly two weeks, which wasn't the way it used to be . . . we were always very active and had a good sex life. But it happened one night when I got undressed and I had this lacy top on. He really got turned on, and we made love. It was great.

"Then he said how hard it was for him to know what I wanted . . . and he wasn't sure about himself either. We talked that night, about sex and about lots of things. Not only didn't he reject me, but we got closer than we'd ever been. We talked about things we'd never talked about before. We've grown closer."

Pam's husband, John, talked about that critical time in a separate interview some months later. An open and frank man, he was very willing to share his thoughts and feelings about Pam's illness and how it affected both of them. "The worst time was when we were waiting for the diagnosis," said John. "And then, I had to tell Pam . . . that was the worst of it. After that, it seemed easy.

"When Pam came back after the mastectomy, I wasn't sure about how to react. I knew she was uptight about the mastectomy, and she didn't want me to see it. To tell you the truth, I wasn't sure about it, and I didn't want to see it either. I'm not sure if it was because I knew she hated that scar or because I just didn't want to see it. But it didn't affect me. I'm a very sexual person, and my desire for her has always been high. It stayed the same. I can't say I ever had any doubts about wanting her . . . physically or otherwise.

"There was that first week or two when I didn't know how to handle it. I didn't want to be insensitive about her feelings, but I didn't want her to come to any wrong conclusions. I held back for a while . . . and now, I think that was probably a mistake. But that's all right. Nature took its course."

Pam's experience was not unusual. If a woman places a great premium on her breast, she may expect her partner to do the same. This may involve the couple's sexual life and their life at large. A woman may fear she will be completely rejected, that her husband won't want to live with a one-breasted woman, and to protect herself, she may withdraw. Her partner may pick up on this distance and respond in kind. It can all become a self-fulfilling prophecy. Or her partner may not wish to reject her but may be much more fearful that she may die. And this may not come to light. Again, failing to communicate with each other is the biggest problem of all.

Men are usually less concerned with the physical and sexual meanings of breast loss than women expect them to be. Instead, most men are much more concerned with the possibility of losing someone they love. Many of our women patients have told us their husbands have been more thankful that their wives were alive and well than they were concerned about the effects of disfigurement. Of course, this may sometimes be a whitewashing of some very profound feelings on the man's part, but every situation has its own individual meanings. The option of breast reconstruction can change a good deal of this equation for the better. It can minimize or eliminate the issue of breast loss. It may prove to be an important component in the overall treatment of a woman *and* her partner when they are *both* coping with breast cancer.

A good marriage not only will survive breast cancer but may very well improve. Some marriages, though, don't survive. A troubled marriage may become more difficult and may even dissolve, but that may more reflect the couple's prior relationship than it does the effects of breast cancer.

🌺 Lucille Greene put it this way:

"I have four friends who've had breast cancer. Two of them are now divorced. A few years ago I'd have been naive enough to blame it on the disease. I'd have thought their marriages broke up *because* of the breast cancer . . . that it affected the marriage.

"Yes, there *was* stress, but those marriages were in trouble *before* that lump was discovered. The relationships couldn't withstand the stress. One friend . . . her husband just withdrew. She was devastated; she felt totally rejected. It turned out that her husband was having an affair all along . . . for three years before she discovered she had breast cancer!

"And the other marriage . . . we all knew it was on shaky grounds for years. It never stood a chance, *with or without* breast cancer. Something like breast cancer doesn't happen in a vacuum; it's a two-way street between a man and a woman. A lot depends on how they've handled things before. It depends on the relationship."

Lucille went on to describe the trouble she and her husband, Bob, had dealing with her illness and the effects it had on their sexual life together.

"Before my surgery and the chemotherapy, Bob never had any sexual problems. There were never any failures. When I first got back from the hospital I had chemotherapy and then radiation. I wasn't at all interested in sex. We didn't have any relations for at least three months. Bob was very loving and caring. He'd caress me and hold me and tell me how much he loved me. It was very important. I can't say I felt he was being rejecting or that he had no sexual interest.

"I didn't notice it for a long time because I was having such a hard time with the chemotherapy, but when the side effects began wearing off, I got interested in sex again. But something had happened . . . to us, to Bob . . . I wasn't sure. He wasn't interested anymore. He was still loving and warm, but he didn't get aroused, no matter what I did.

"I knew he had a problem now, a problem that wasn't there before the breast cancer. Maybe it's better to say *we* had a problem at that point, because I was getting a little frustrated. We let it go on for a long time without saying anything, without confronting the problem, but we finally talked about it. Bob cried and said he didn't know what was wrong, that something had changed but he didn't know what it was. My having breast cancer affected us both, and he didn't know what happened to his sex drive. It was gone.

"It's been three years now and we began getting counseling a few months ago. So far there's been no change. It's still a problem, but we're talking about it, and about other things too. It's silly to pretend my cancer and the treatments didn't affect us, it did. But we're working on it."

Some men become oversolicitous. They may treat a woman as though she's suddenly become an invalid. One patient told us that her husband suddenly began catering to her. He wanted to hire a housekeeper and would barely let his wife do anything by herself. "He finally calmed down when I told him he was making me feel like a terminal case!" the patient said.

Some men try to be overly reassuring. Words such as *It's nothing . . . don't worry . . .* imply that the woman is exaggerating the seriousness of her condition, that it doesn't warrant deep concern. This can be a subtle message that a woman may have to bear her emotional burden alone, that her partner doesn't want to hear about it.

Men often have as many worries, fears, anxieties, and questions about breast cancer and mastectomy as their partners do. For this reason, some men find it helpful to get involved in group sessions along with their partners, although this is not for everyone. Many men have trouble acknowledging to themselves or to others that they have feelings and needs. If this is the case, a man is probably better off trying to deal with his feelings away from the pressure of a group setting.

Many women—and men too—are very concerned about their sexuality following the diagnosis and treatment of breast cancer. This is especially true for women and their partners if there has been a mastectomy without reconstruction. If your husband thinks you are weak or not ready for intercourse, he will be understandably reluctant to approach you. This can confirm your own fears of rejection. Again, failure to communicate (on many levels) is the biggest problem.

For some couples, the earlier intercourse takes place after the woman's arrival home, the better the situation will be. Pam's husband, John, seemed to recognize that when he reflected back on that 2-week period of time after Pam came home. He was uncertain about how to react, and he waited for "nature" to take its course. In some situations, a woman may not feel physically or emotionally ready for intercourse. Each should take cues from the other, but remember, when something as emotionally charged as your sexual life depends only on cues, there may be silent misunderstanding.

If you and your partner can share your thoughts and feelings about the changes in your lives at this time, you may find yourselves developing a new closeness. Your awareness of each other may actually heighten everything for both of you—your openness, your closeness, and your sensitivity toward each other.

🌺 Carol Collins was 40 years old when she learned she had breast cancer. You may recall that her initial reaction was grave concern for her son, whom she and her husband had adopted after a long struggle. A few years later she reflected back on how her life had changed since that day the diagnosis was made.

"My having breast cancer changed me and Phillip [her husband]. We learned a lot about each other and about ourselves. Sexually, it was very rough . . . we were both unsure about where it would go. And I'm still not sure because we've never quite gotten our sexual life back on track.

"But there are other things. If I really admit it to myself,

I was never that sure about Phillip's really loving me. I mean, I knew he cared and when we adopted our son it was a tremendous commitment, one I wasn't sure Phillip could make. In all truth, I always doubted Phillip's commitment . . . until I got through the breast cancer. Maybe I should say after *we* got through it together, because that's what it was—something we went through together.

"Sexually, we aren't as good as we once were. But we're much closer now. And overall, I think we're better than we ever were with each other."

Single or divorced women have other difficulties to deal with. These women often ask when a man should be told about their having had breast cancer. Or when should they tell him about their mastectomy?

There is no rule for this kind of thing. Some women feel very comfortable talking about it right away; others feel they must wait until a certain level of intimacy has already been established.

🌺 Diana Benson was a 46-year-old woman who had had a mastectomy 3 years earlier. She was divorced, lived alone in New York City, and was a successful executive at an advertising agency. She talked frankly about her life and her relationships:

"As far as telling a man . . . for me, it's easy. I tell him right at the beginning. I don't waste any time. Maybe it's defensive, but I don't want to get involved—especially a physical thing—and get emotionally tangled up with a man and then drop this *bomb* on his head! Because then, it's hard to know . . . is he sticking around out of pity? Because he feels obligated? Too embarrassed to pick up and go? Who knows? This way, on the first date, when we meet, I mention it casually, like you might mention having an appendectomy a few years ago, and I let it go from there. Some men don't seem to mind; others . . . you never hear from them again. But you don't necessarily know why. I can't waste time worrying about it. After all, it's hard enough being 46 and alone."

🌿 Susan Miller was a 39-year-old stockbroker. Separated for 2 years, she dealt with this concern in a different way. She felt that telling too soon may load the dice unfavorably.

"For me, I've got to feel I know a man pretty well. We've got to be getting closer and I've got to feel we'll be sexually intimate soon. Otherwise, why tell? It'll only push something before it's ready and I don't feel that's fair, for either of us."

When Susan was about to have a reconstruction, she thought that her physical situation would change, although other things would remain debatable.

"I know the physical thing—my having one breast—will change for the better, but there's still the whole thing about telling a man you've had *cancer.* Some men can never handle it—they might just as well hear you've got leprosy—but that's no loss. In the long run, you've got to find your own way . . . with the disease, with yourself, and maybe with the right man."

The single or divorced woman with one breast may find the option of breast reconstruction especially valuable. Here, where there may not be a long-term emotional involvement with a committed partner and where there is the understandable concern about how a new man may react, a woman may strongly feel she wants her lost breast replaced. We will discuss this aspect of breast surgery in the next chapter.

As is true with your relationship in general, your sexual life with your partner will be an extension of your situation prior to the diagnosis and treatment for breast cancer. The chances are that if things went well before this time, they will continue the same way, providing you and your partner communicate. If each of you can keep in touch with your own feelings, and if you can share them with each other, you can build on whatever was in the relationship. This may bring richness and greater compatibility, both sexually and in your lives at large.

However, it would be naive to expect no troubles. Even the most sympathetic partners will have misunderstandings. You and your partner must make important adjustments, individually and together, and this is rarely easy. Expect that each of you will have periods of moodiness. Expect occasional moments of insensitivity from your partner. There will most likely be difficulties, frustration, tears, and moments of anger, just as there would be in your life anyway. However, because of your illness and its implications, these may take on a sharper focus and have more impact than they otherwise would.

Remember too that your having had breast cancer may evoke in your partner some of *his* own childhood fears and fantasies. Your husband may ordinarily take illness and other family difficulties in stride, but there may have been a distant relative he dimly recalls who died of cancer years ago. You may not know how your illness affects your partner on a variety of levels.

Still, if you have a solid relationship that has worked well in the past, it is unlikely that this family crisis will drag your marriage into deeply troubled waters. In our experience, with the proper communication in a relationship that has

worked all along, both partners eventually feel they traveled
a difficult course but emerged feeling closer, more committed, and more loving than before.

What do I tell my children? How do I tell them?

Many parents wonder if they should tell children when
their mother develops breast cancer. While there may be
occasional exceptions, the general rule of thumb is very clear:
Your children should know what is going on. As most parents
know, children are amazingly perceptive; they sense when
something is wrong or different in the family or with either
parent. A very young child may conjure up the most frightening fantasies to explain your absence or a change in your
behavior.

When you return home, your child will clearly sense that
something is different. If the child is left with the vagueness
of his or her fantasies, the situation may assume terrifying
proportions.

On the other hand, there is no rule about *how* or *when*
to tell a child. Some children will become frightened by a
visit to the hospital; others may feel reassured seeing that
you are well and knowing you will return home in a few
days.

To prepare yourself for the discussion with your children,
you and your husband might think up the various questions
you expect your child to have about the illness and the
family situation. If you are having radiotherapy or chemotherapy, visits to the hospital will have to be explained to
the preschool child. Any meaningful change in your routines
should be explained in simple, clear terms that your child
can understand.

You and your husband should also remember that your
child may have many questions about the illness, but may
not express them all. Prepare yourself to answer these ques-

tions too: What other treatments will you need? Will you sometimes feel sick? Will you be upset and sad?

Certainly, your responses to questions will depend on your child's age and capacity to understand your situation. Adolescent children may have special difficulty dealing with cancer and the emotional issues it brings up in the family. Adolescence is often filled with turmoil. It is not unusual to see bewildering behavior changes. These may include drinking, promiscuity, sullenness, and a range of behaviors all resulting from the young adult's being drawn back into the family when he or she was beginning to separate from the parents and to look beyond the home.

If you have a teenage daughter, she may need additional attention. She may wonder if she will someday develop breast cancer herself. Again, silence will not alleviate unnecessary or exaggerated fears. A frank discussion with your daughter about her increased risk will be helpful. You should explain the crucial importance of practicing regular breast self-examination and of having regular breast examinations by a physician. This family crisis may provide you and your daughter with an extraordinary chance to grow closer.

Naturally, children of any age will respond to your illness within the context of their own maturity and of the family relationships. However, one thing is very clear: The unknown is almost always more frightening than the reality, whether you are dealing with your own reactions to breast cancer or those of your husband and children.

What about my job? How will my coworkers react to me and my illness? What can I expect when I return?

A working woman who has been treated for breast cancer may have to make other adjustments in addition to returning to her family. Most women wish to return to work at some point; they are eager to pick up the threads of their personal and work lives. An understandable concern is how others will react to them when they return.

Unfortunately, your returning to work may not always be greeted with enthusiasm. If you have been out for a substantial period of time, your employer may have been given enough information about your hospital course to know you have been treated for cancer. This can work negatively in some job situations. Many people still think that someone with cancer is terminal. Job discrimination, when it occurs, orbits around the myth that someone with cancer, of any kind, is sick, will continue to be sick, and will be an unreliable employee.

Studies conducted 12 years ago by the Metropolitan Life Insurance Company concluded that employees treated for cancer had the same level of performance, the same job turnover rate, and the same number of absences as did other workers. Still, many employers are reluctant to rehire someone who, in their view, has had a potentially fatal illness.

Then there is the question of insurance coverage. Many small businesses are reluctant to hire people who could send insurance premiums skyrocketing, since a federal law states that all employees must have equal insurance benefits. At the present time, so far as we know, no progress has been made in getting the federal government to pay for the insurance of workers who have had a long-term or catastrophic illness. We certainly hope a more enlightened approach will be adopted in the very near future.

Most breast cancer patients who return to work seem to agree that the relationship with an employer (boss, supervisor, management personnel in general) is much easier and smoother if an employee has been with the company for a long time and has had a reliable work record.

If you are a professional woman, you may have more flexibility than a salaried worker with fairly routine hours. This can be helpful if you are having chemotherapy, which may seriously impede a smooth transition back to work. You may be forced to miss occasional days, and your job performance may be affected. Obviously, this is something you need to have cleared with your employer before returning to work. A radiation schedule may involve commuting or even temporarily relocating near the facility, which may delay your return to work.

❧ Many women wonder about the reactions of colleagues when they return to work. Teacher Barbara Conti said:

"It was 12 years ago and I think attitudes were different then; I'm not sure. But there was a lot of silence. It was clear that no one was going to talk about it unless I brought it up, and even then, I detected a lot of reluctance. I had a structured workday, and much of my time was with the kids. That shielded me. After a while, it became a peripheral issue. After all these years, I don't think anyone knows or even cares."

❧ Pam Reimer felt acutely anxious and self-conscious when she returned to work at the law firm.

"I just told people I'd had breast surgery," she said, recalling that time a year later. "I didn't get specific. I never mentioned 'cancer' to anyone and I don't really know if they ever knew. But *I* knew and sometimes I would wonder if anyone was staring and trying to figure which breast it was . . . women, men . . . it didn't matter. The only ones I told were two good friends. It was like I had this terrible secret."

* * *

Pam's sense of secrecy is not unusual. Many returning breast cancer patients fear that coworkers will snub them. Some fellow employees may even think cancer is contagious. For some people there may be a stigma attached to the word *cancer*. This may partly be because people don't know how to deal with someone who has been seriously ill. Some people feel very uncomfortable being around a person who they fear may die. For other coworkers, the presence of someone who has had cancer may force them to face an uncomfortable reminder of human vulnerability, especially their own.

The only rule of thumb we would apply to telling coworkers is to think carefully about whom you may wish to tell. You might want to tell someone toward whom you feel a closeness, or you may not. Some people may surprise you with their openness and supportiveness. Others may keep some distance. Remember, coworkers will respond to your having breast cancer in the context of their own lives, their own problems, their own fantasies, and their own expectations from childhood. It's a complicated issue for most people. Knowing that, you may then choose whom to tell about your experience.

Some patients have told us that after returning to work or to their normal routines, they feel that some people expect them to adopt the role of a "nobly dying patient." It is difficult to know if this is true or if it is an inner feeling that some patients have about themselves and that they project onto others. Undoubtedly, certain people, when faced with someone who has cancer, will unwittingly convey the unspoken (and sometimes spoken) expectation that the person will die.

Such attitudes are formed by popular myth, by long-standing social stereotypes, and by the various media treatments of cancer. (The films *Love Story* and *Terms of Endearment* are only two of many films over the years that have portrayed cancer as a fatal disease.) Simply knowing that some people will react this way may be helpful.

Remember, you cannot change people's deeply rooted fears, prejudices, and misconceptions. You can only deal with your own thoughts, feelings, and expectations.

How will friends react? Whom should I tell?

Friends, too, will react to your illness in the context of their lives, both past and present—and in the context of your friendship. Many women we have seen with breast cancer have already had one or two friends who developed the disease. Others have often formed a relationship with someone else whose circumstances are similar. But don't feel you must exclusively stick to such relationships. Just as with those closest to you, a good friend will make psychological adjustments to your situation and will deal with it as another facet of the relationship. In the long run, breast cancer, like any life crisis, tests the mettle of those close to you. Your dearest friends are no exception.

What about the beach? How will my wardrobe be changed?

These are serious cosmetic considerations. Many women find the daily routine of wearing a prosthesis or of making allowances for certain clothing a constant reminder of breast cancer. Today, with less extensive surgery you have choices never available in the days when the standard operation was the Halsted radical mastectomy. And the option of breast reconstruction now makes many of these cosmetic issues virtually obsolete.

Am I neurotic for thinking about breast reconstruction? Shouldn't I be thankful I'm alive and not even think about it? Am I being vain? Am I too old for it?

These are some of the questions we hear about breast reconstruction. The answer to most of them is, No! Today, you can have breast reconstruction after a mastectomy. And you can have excellent results. This can eliminate the psychological adjustment for the woman who has a mastectomy and who must then spend years coping with feelings about having one breast. In the past, women did not have this option, since plastic surgeons have only recently perfected new techniques and the general public only now is becoming aware of it. But there are many women who had mastectomies 5, 10, or more years ago who may be excellent candidates for breast reconstruction today.

Of course, this step is not for every woman, but it can be enormously helpful for many. It is a quality-of-life decision. There is nothing vain or neurotic about wishing to appear as you did before you became ill. There is nothing selfish or narcissistic about wishing to appear normal, even when you are undressed. Some doctors express surprise when they encounter an older woman interested in having a breast reconstructed. The feeling *you're too old for this* is a kind of bias, since it assumes older people have no interest in sexual matters or appearance. And besides, a woman's wish for reconstruction is not exclusively sexual.

We have already discussed the crucial importance of body image and how it enters into your view of yourself as a person, a woman, and a mother. Breast reconstruction is solidly bound to seeing yourself as normal, healthy, and whole.

TEN

Breast Reconstruction

Today, more and more women are expressing interest in breast reconstruction to replace their missing breasts. There are a number of forces at work in this emerging trend. For one thing, early detection techniques are resulting in more women with smaller breast lumps coming for treatment. Along with this has been the trend toward less extensive surgery in the treatment of breast cancer. These two factors mean that there are more women who are better candidates for reconstruction now than there were when Halsted radical mastectomy was the main treatment. With minimal surgery and radiation, there is often no need for reconstruction, although this is not always the case. The location of certain lumps may mean their removal will result in extensive deformity, and if the patient wishes to return to a normal appearance, reconstruction will be required.

Through articles in popular magazines and newspapers, the general public is becoming more aware and more accepting of reconstruction after breast surgery. More general surgeons, too, are becoming aware of breast reconstruction, whereas a few years ago many surgeons, concerned mainly with eradicating the tumor, never mentioned the possibility of reconstruction to their patients. As a matter of fact, a National Cancer Institute poll taken 10 years ago showed that only one-quarter of the women polled were even *aware of the option of reconstruction* after having a mastectomy. This has certainly changed.

Today, women are taking a more active role in their health and well-being and are requesting information about reconstruction from their physicians. Indeed, they often choose physicians who know about breast reconstruction, who favor such surgery, and who are willing to consult with a plastic surgeon even before a mastectomy is done. The presence of a reconstructive surgeon as part of a treatment team is important to many patients. Having information about reconstruction as soon as possible may lighten the emotional impact of mastectomy and it may give the patient the feeling that she is actively making treatment plans for her future.

Another important reason why breast reconstruction is more commonly done is that plastic surgeons have developed new and innovative techniques. Years ago, with the radical mastectomy, it was difficult to simulate a missing breast. The results often left a great deal to be desired and were achieved only by a long and arduous series of operations. As in many other areas of medicine, advances have been made in plastic and reconstructive surgery so more consistent and cosmetically pleasing results are generally obtained.

Perhaps most important has been the tendency for women to place emphasis on the quality of their lives after mastectomy. All patients are concerned about losing a breast, regardless of its size or shape. A scar on a woman's chest is often as much a psychological scar as it is a physical phenomenon. It is a constant reminder of the disease. An external prosthesis may be another constant reminder. Many women report feeling uncomfortable wearing these devices. It requires constant concern and adjustment and never becomes part of a woman's body image. And no matter how well the device looks when a woman is fully dressed, it doesn't provide any semblance of a normal appearance in sexual relationships.

The proprietor of a shop specializing in postmastectomy apparel said, "All my clients are unwilling customers, and over 90 percent are dissatisfied with the best-fitting prostheses we can provide."* Special precautions must be taken with certain styles of clothing. Some swimwear and sportswear will not work with a prosthesis. For many women this is a frustrating and life-limiting reminder of deformity and disease.

Above all, it is the psychological concern about the integrity of her body and the way she feels about herself that brings a woman to a plastic surgeon for reconstruction. For many women, breast reconstruction is part of a total program of physical, social, and emotional rehabilitation. It may be the first concrete step a woman takes *beyond* her breast cancer and the sense of loss and fear this disease evokes.

Having seen many women during various phases of their encounters with breast cancer, we have concluded that for many, the decision to have reconstructive breast surgery is as much a decision to restore and reconstruct themselves emotionally as it is a decision to rebuild a breast. Knowing she can have breast reconstruction can change a woman's

---

* Quoted in E. Anstice, "Coping after Mastectomy," *Nursing Times* 66 (1970): 882–83.

entire experience and her expectations of breast cancer. It can lessen the disease's impact on her life and on her options. It can enhance the feeling of having some element of control over the events in her life. Many women report feeling less "victimized" by breast cancer, knowing they can restore this vital body part.

In our opinion, the option of breast reconstruction should be known by every woman before any treatment method is begun. Reconstruction should be considered an integral part of the treatment of breast cancer, even as the disease is being diagnosed and a treatment plan is being formulated. This does not mean every woman will want it or have it. But it should be an option that is discussed by a woman and her physician, even before a decision is made about which treatment will work best for her. This part of a team approach to the treatment of breast cancer takes into account the needs of the whole person, physically, cosmetically, and emotionally.

Women's profound concerns about the impact of breast surgery are now being recognized and are influencing the way breast cancer is being treated. Insurance companies are now classifying breast reconstruction as rehabilitative surgery, *not* as cosmetic surgery. As a result, most major medical insurance policies cover breast reconstruction in their plans.

Ideally, the surgeon's function is to rid the patient of her disease and to restore her physical and psychological well-being. Over the years, surgeons have removed breasts and often rid the patient of her disease. However, the second half of this goal was rarely considered. Breast reconstruction is now recognized as contributing to *that* other half of the goal.

There is little doubt that breast reconstruction will become even more accepted by the general public and the medical profession at large. Many plastic surgeons feel strongly that once women are more aware of this surgery as a real option in the treatment of breast cancer, they may be more willing to make a life-saving visit to a doctor when they discover symptoms of the disease.

Who Is a Candidate for Breast Reconstruction?

Before you can have a breast reconstruction, your plastic surgeon will carefully consider your individual case history. Many plastic surgeons feel that the best candidates for reconstruction are women who have had small tumors (less than 2 centimeters) and who have had less than three positive lymph nodes found in the axilla. Other surgeons maintain that virtually any woman who has had breast cancer should be able to have her breast rebuilt if she chooses to do so. There are different techniques for rebuilding the breast depending on the extent of surgery a woman has had. Each patient must be considered on an individual basis.

A prime concern of any plastic surgeon is a patient's motivation for wanting her breast rebuilt. Women requesting the operation are usually motivated by a healthy desire to feel more comfortable and to have fewer restrictions on the clothing they can wear. They are also motivated by the need to feel whole again, to remove that "space" that is a constant reminder of breast loss and of disease, and to feel they are regaining some control over their lives.

Some patients, however, have inappropriate motives for breast reconstruction. Rebuilding your breast will not erase the fact that you have had breast cancer. It will not magically eradicate the disease, and it will not reduce the need for constant follow-up in both the affected breast and the opposite one. Breast reconstruction will not solve other problems in life; if you and your partner are having difficulties, a rebuilt breast will not soothe troubles away. It will not restore a lost love affair or rebuild a crumbling marriage. It is not a passport to a new way of life after having breast cancer.

Sometimes, too, a patient may not be motivated at all for breast reconstruction.

❧ Mary Rossi and her husband came to the plastic surgeon's office requesting a consultation about the possibility of reconstructing Mrs. Rossi's breast. It had been removed 11 years earlier when she was 50 years old because of a small tumor that had proved to be cancerous.

During their discussion, it became clear to the surgeon that Mrs. Rossi was quite satisfied with her prosthesis and with the way things had gone in her life since her treatment for breast cancer. She had accepted having one breast, and it had not been a problem since her operation. The Rossis' lives had gone well, and they still had an active sexual life together.

In fact, Mrs. Rossi had no particular interest in having another operation. She sought out the plastic surgeon because her cousin had repeatedly urged her to do so. The couple had come for the consultation only to "find out" about this operation. The motivation was entirely missing. For Mrs. Rossi, having survived the diagnosis and treatment was sufficient. Her individual needs were satisfied, and she was not a good candidate for breast reconstruction.

One of the most important tasks of your plastic surgeon is to help you recognize preoperatively what can and cannot be accomplished by breast reconstruction. The only way to do this is by showing you pre- and postoperative photographs of other patients who have undergone similar procedures. They should be women who are of similar stature and have similar breast configuration and skin tone to yours.

Many women have frightening fantasies of the destruction caused by mastectomy. Very few have a working idea about the quality today's reconstructive techniques can achieve in restoring the breast contours to normal. Photographic aids can effectively bring these issues into focus.

When to Have a Breast Rebuilt

There is no single best time for having breast reconstruction. If your tumor is small and requires minimal surgery, many plastic surgeons prefer combining reconstruction with the mastectomy. They feel that most women want reconstruction as soon as possible; waiting 6 months or a year, or longer, does not always take the patient's wishes into account. By combining the procedures, much of the trauma of mastectomy is alleviated since the patient comes out of the operation having already begun her rehabilitation. This can be a very important psychological plus. Surgeons also feel that combining the procedures makes the reconstruction less costly. The plastic surgeon works with the general surgeon during the operation.

Other plastic surgeons prefer to wait for a period of 3 months to 1 year after mastectomy so that the wound heals completely. Waiting also allows the transfer of your care from the general surgeon who removed the cancer to the plastic surgeon who will reconstruct your breast. In some instances, there can be a team approach. During your cancer surgery both surgeons can work together so the incision can be positioned for minimal scar formation. This requires greater coordination between your treating physicians, and it provides the best possible care for you.

Even if radiotherapy and chemotherapy are important parts of your overall treatment plan, reconstruction is still possible and need not interfere with your other treatment. The timing of the reconstructive procedures may have to be adjusted to your specific needs, but reconstruction can be performed.

The time of your consultation for breast reconstruction is important. Ideally, it should occur before your mastectomy, during your pre-operative workup, so you can consider all the options. This can help you feel that although you are about to face treatment for breast cancer, you are also undertaking a course of rehabilitation. However, some women are so upset and anxious when entering the hospital for their initial breast surgery, they cannot think about breast reconstruction. Whether your consultation with a plastic surgeon occurs before or after your breast surgery, you should have a frank and complete discussion of your situation. Do not be surprised if your plastic surgeon asks why you want reconstruction or if the question comes up about your hopes and expectations of this surgery.

Again, pre- and postoperative photographs of other patients before *your* cancer surgery can be very helpful. This can help you develop a better mental image of what you yourself may look like, both after your mastectomy and after your subsequent breast reconstruction. These mental images, based on the reality of other patients' results, can be a source of well-founded optimism at a difficult time. More than one patient has said that knowing she could eventually look normal again made a mastectomy itself more tolerable.

Regardless of the timing of your consultation with a plastic surgeon, he or she may want to consult with the surgeon doing the mastectomy or lumpectomy to help get a firm idea of your medical situation. This would also allow the plastic surgeon to suggest certain technical considerations to your surgeon that, if possible in your case, could mean easier reconstruction. All this depends on the location and size of your tumor and on the exchange of information between your surgeons.

Techniques of Reconstruction

The method of breast reconstruction your plastic surgeon uses will depend on the extent of your mastectomy surgery. It will also take into account your body weight and the size, shape, and position of your remaining breast. The reconstruction involves two basic processes: rebuilding the breast mound and rebuilding the areola and nipple.

Rebuilding the Mound

TISSUE TRANSFER

There are several ways to reconstruct the lost bulk of the breast tissue, the surrounding fat as well as the overlying skin. First, tissue may be brought from other areas. This can be done in several ways. Any transported tissue will require that a good blood supply be maintained if it is to remain viable. Local tissue, that is, tissue located adjacent to the deformity, may serve as a source of reconstructive tissue when minimal surgery has been done. At times, local skin flaps may be all that is required to nicely reconstruct the defect in the breast.

There are areas nearby where tissue may be lifted but left attached to its own blood supply and moved to the breast area. This kind of transfer is called a muscle-skin flap, since muscle, skin, and intervening fat are all transferred. There are presently two areas commonly used to supply tissue for this type of reconstruction. One is the back, immediately behind the missing breast on the same side, called the latissimus-dorsi flap. The other donor site is the lower part of the abdomen.

In the latissimus-dorsi flap method, an artificial silicone implant is usually needed to add sufficient bulk to the transplant. The vertical scar from the donor site is situated on the back. There is also a slight defect beneath the skin due to absent muscle on this side. Nevertheless, there is usually very little decrease in shoulder function.

In the abdominal donor-site operation there is usually sufficient fat and skin so that a prosthesis is not necessary. With this technique, the scar at the donor site is positioned across the abdomen, usually below the level of the umbilicus, and is therefore easily hidden with clothing. The muscle taken from the abdomen in the transfer of the flap may slightly weaken the abdominal wall from which it was removed. Special attention is sometimes necessary to ensure that an abdominal hernia does not occur after the tissue transfer.

These tissue transfer techniques can bring in vital tissue to rebuild large defects where a breast was totally removed. Some radical mastectomy patients who have had removal of the chest wall muscles along with the breast may have very adequate breast reconstruction with these methods. These techniques are also important for patients who have had extensive skin damage after having radiotherapy treatments. The amount of bulk needed for reconstruction is of course an individual decision depending largely on the condition of the opposite breast. We will have more to say about this later.

Another method of bringing the patient's own tissue into the area of reconstruction requires microvascular techniques of surgery. Muscle and overlying fat and skin are transferred by cutting the main blood vessels of the donor site area and reconnecting them to adequate blood vessels of the breast area. In this type of operation the flap is "free" from the body during the transfer and, therefore, the method is called free-flap. This allows the surgeon to select a donor site farther from the breast. An excellent choice is the buttock area. At this site there is usually adequate tissue for rebuilding the lost bulk, and the scars can easily be hidden. The techniques required for a microvascular transfer are more complicated than with other techniques and are therefore less commonly done.

TISSUE EXPANSION AND BREAST PROSTHESES

The breast mound may also be simulated through the use of prostheses alone. This method takes into account the ability of local skin and muscle to be gradually stretched. If the skin was suddenly stretched, its blood supply could collapse under the pressure of the stretching and skin death would result.

When people gain or lose weight, their skin stretches and shrinks as the underlying volume gradually increases and decreases. This talent of skin—its stretchability over a period of time—is exploited by tissue expansion techniques.

An inflatable silicone bladder is inserted under the skin and, often, under the muscle of the chest wall where the breast is to be reconstructed. This bladder is connected by tubing to a buttonlike reservoir that is implanted just below the skin. Once the bladder is in place, at subsequent office visits, the physician injects salt water solution through the skin into the reservoir, thereby increasing the volume of the silicone bladder. This allows for a gradual stretching of the overlying skin and muscle over a period of several weeks. When adequate volume is obtained, slightly more solution is added to further stretch the overlying skin and muscle. This slight "overstretching" allows for a more natural-looking final result.

Finally, the bladder-expander is removed, and the final prosthesis is substituted into the surgically created pocket. This exchange of implants is a relatively minor procedure and may be done under local anesthesia on an out-patient basis.

Sometimes, when the plastic surgeon is simulating a small breast, the final prosthesis may be implanted during the initial procedure, when the pocket is surgically created. This of course depends on the volume that must be simulated and on the condition of the overlying skin and muscle.

Several types of silicone prostheses have been used for the last 25 years, and in all that time, there has been no reported incidence of their ever causing breast cancer. No additional scars of the chest wall or other areas of the body need be made. The operation is less time-consuming than tissue transfer techniques, and in properly selected patients, the cosmetic results are excellent.

POSSIBLE COMPLICATIONS

With any surgical intervention into the body's workings, there is always the chance of complications. The following are the occasional complications of surgery where the breast mound is reconstructed:

WITH TISSUE TRANSFER

- Excessive bleeding at the operative site. This rarely causes severe problems.
- Infection. The rate of infection in these procedures is low. If it occurs, it can be treated with antibiotics.
- Loss of blood supply to the transferred tissue. With the

transfer of any tissue, the blood supply is all-important. At times, because the blood supply may be compromised, the entire flap or a portion of the flap may die. If this occurs, the dead tissue and the underlying implant (if one is used) must be removed. Further surgery may be necessary to rectify the problem.

WITH TISSUE EXPANSION TECHNIQUES

- Bleeding into the implant pocket. If the amount of blood is excessive, it may require surgical removal.
- Occasionally, infection at the site of the surgery. This can be treated with antibiotics, but if the infection persists, the implant may have to be removed.
- Capsule formation. The body reacts to the silicone implant by forming a scar tissue capsule around the prosthesis. At times, this scar tissue may tighten, making the reconstructed breast very firm to the touch. Any breast reconstructed by an implant technique will feel slightly more firm than a normal breast. Placing the prosthesis beneath both the skin and the muscle of the chest wall makes capsule formation less likely and less noticeable if it does occur. If a hard capsule forms, it can be treated by a surgeon in the office and is a less extensive procedure than the initial operation.

Rebuilding the Nipple and Areola

Once the breast mound has been rebuilt, many patients wish to then have a second, small operation—a nipple and areola reconstruction. There are various techniques to accomplish this.

The opposite nipple and areola not only serve as a model for reconstruction but are frequently sources for reconstructive tissue. The reconstruction is mainly concerned with simulating the color of the areola and the prominence of the nipple of the other breast.

THE NIPPLE

If the nipple on the opposite side is large enough, a portion of it may be taken to provide a graft to the reconstruction site. The goal is to obtain equal nipple prominence on both sides. However, if the opposite nipple is not sufficiently prominent, other sources of tissue are available. The local skin at the site of reconstruction, if adequate, may be elevated by using a series of operative procedures to give the effect of nipple prominence. Grafts from other areas such as the earlobe also serve as excellent sources for nipple reconstruction.

THE AREOLA

The object in areola reconstruction is to match the color and size of the areola on the natural breast. This may be done by taking tissue from the opposite side (if the areola is large enough) and grafting it to the reconstructed side. Grafts from skin behind the ear, groin skin, and labial skin are also excellent sources of tissue for areola reconstruction. Of these various donor sites, the tissue from behind the ear is the lightest in color; the groin skin is more pigmented; the labial skin is still more pigmented. The proper choice of donor site depends on the color of the natural areola.

Sometimes, for greater symmetry, both the areola of the natural breast and of the reconstructed breast may be treated. A portion of the unaffected areola is removed—taking a thin slice with its pigmentation. Donor skin is taken from the inner thigh area and then grafted to both sides. The result is excellent symmetry both in size and color between the natural and the reconstructed areola.

POSSIBLE COMPLICATIONS

Again, with any surgical procedure there may be complications. With nipple and areola reconstruction, the following complications may occur:

- Infection at the operative site. This may be treated with antibiotics.
- Excessive bleeding at the operative site.
- Loss of grafted tissue. When tissue is grafted to a new area, blood vessels must attach to the graft to keep this tissue nourished and alive. At times, owing to infection, bleeding, or displacement of the graft, this hookup does not properly take place. In such an instance, the graft will not survive, and the procedure may have to be repeated.

ABOUT NIPPLE/AREOLA BANKING

No longer in favor or frequently done is nipple and areola banking, a technique that involves saving the nipple/areola complex of the removed breast until it can be replaced on the reconstructed breast at a later time. Before a nipple is banked, it must be carefully checked by a pathologist for any evidence of cancer. Then the nipple is sewn on to the lower abdomen, the usual storage site.

Because there is a chance that the saved nipple may harbor microcolonies of cancer cells, or may later develop cancer, many surgeons feel that nipple banking should not be practiced. Also, from a cosmetic point of view, there is sometimes a loss of color of the saved areola.

Knowing Your Options for Reconstruction

Your plastic and reconstructive surgeon has a repertoire of breast reconstruction techniques. Each technique has a specific application for any given patient depending on her body fat, its distribution, and the condition of the overlying skin, the muscle, and other tissue. Each method of reconstruction has its advantages and drawbacks depending on a patient's specific case. These techniques can be used to full advantage only when a patient with her individual requirements and emotional concerns is fully evaluated and has had a chance to explore her alternatives.

Knowing about your options for breast reconstruction should make you less fearful of the possibility of deformity. This means you should be more willing to self-examine and come for treatment should you discover a lump. This could save your life.

The Other Breast

If you had a mastectomy and are having reconstruction of your breast, you must also decide on your aesthetic goals. If the remaining natural breast is very large or too low, you may wish to consider surgery of this breast so that it matches your reconstructed breast. Plastic and reconstructive surgeons have performed such operations for many years. From teenagers with massive breast development to older women with extremely sagging breasts, many women have chosen this operation to decrease breast size or to elevate breasts to their former position.

In addition to aesthetic considerations, there may be concern about cancer possibly occurring in the other breast. If so, the cosmetic purpose of reconstruction may be *combined* with the treatment program to reduce this risk by having reconstruction of the affected breast along with a subcutaneous mastectomy of the opposite breast. (See Chapter 6, page 110, "The Other Breast.")

After the Operation

The postoperative recuperative period after breast reconstruction will vary depending on the type of procedure done.
With tissue transfer techniques, several days of hospitalization are usually the rule. The incisions at the donor site as
well as in the area of the breast reconstruction will require
some care and observation. Patients having breast reconstruction done with tissue expansion and prostheses often
return home the day after surgery. A series of follow-up
visits is usually made to observe the healing process.

A number of years ago when breast reconstruction techniques were first being developed, cosmetic results were not
always as gratifying as patients and their surgeons would
have liked. However, recent developments in implant methods and innovative surgical techniques for breast mound
and for nipple/areola reconstruction have greatly improved
reconstruction so that the cosmetic results are generally excellent.

❧ Pam Reimer underwent breast reconstruction a year
after her mastectomy. Pam had known all along that she
would have her breast reconstructed, and she had a great
deal to say about this decision.

"My husband knew I wanted a new breast even before I
had my surgery. He said over and over that it wasn't
important to him, that I didn't have to have it, but that if
I wanted it, he was behind me all the way. It was important
to *me,* and it was even more important *after* the mastectomy.
When I'd look in the mirror, I would hate myself . . . hate
the way I *looked.* I couldn't wait until my surgeon gave
me the green light. What was most important to me was
that *I* knew I didn't have two breasts, and then there was

the whole thing about wearing sexy clothes. So I can't kid myself—I did it for myself, and I did it so I could be seen just like any other normal woman. It was important for me not to feel different."

Pam had her reconstruction. She also chose to have a subcutaneous mastectomy and insertion of an implant in her opposite breast—to combine her reconstruction along with a recontouring of her opposite breast and, at the same time, reduce the possibility of developing a second tumor at some time in the future. (See photographs on pages 183, 184, and 185.)

"I decided to give myself a present," Pam said after talking about this decision. "I asked Dr. Cirillo to give me a little bit extra . . . in each breast, you know? Why not? After what I'd been through, it was good to feel I had some say in what happened to me."

🌣 Barbara Conti told about making her decision 12 years after her mastectomy.

"I can't say it was a burning issue, but there was this nagging feeling I couldn't get rid of. A feeling that no matter what, I wasn't the way a woman should be. I'd gotten used to having only one breast, and I'd forget about it for days at a time. But every now and then, the fact of it would stare me in the face. I think that after the initial trauma of it, after the first year or two, I rationalized a lot of it away. I can't really say I adjusted.

"I'm not a vain person. I've never been a beauty queen, and I never placed a premium on my looks. I'd say that for the most part I considered myself fairly plain . . . but I was normal. With one breast missing, I couldn't feel I was

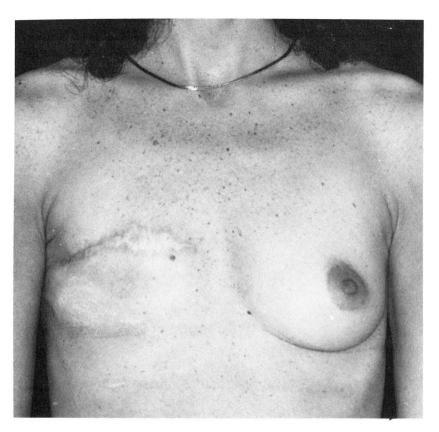

Pam Reimer is shown 6 months after having had her right breast removed by a modified radical mastectomy. Her scar could have been less obvious had more consideration been given to reconstruction at the time of her mastectomy. These concerns can best be dealt with by a team approach where a general surgeon and a plastic surgeon are involved in the treatment program. This helps assure that the patient's cosmetic and emotional needs are taken into account.

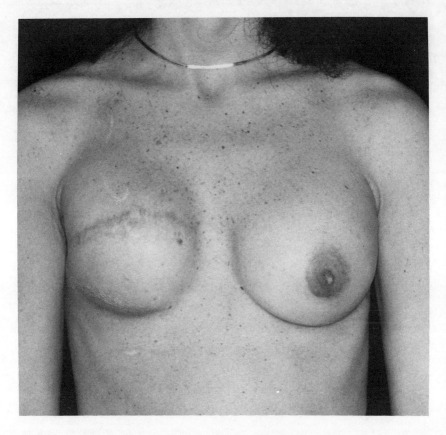

Some months later, Pam had her right breast mound rebuilt with a silicone implant. She also chose to have a subcutaneous mastectomy of her left breast, which was done along with the insertion of an implant. She chose to have her breasts slightly enlarged.

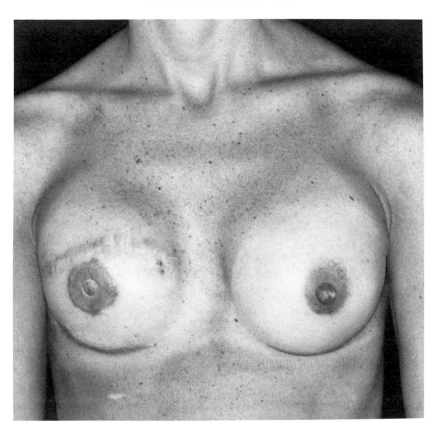

One year after her mastectomy, Pam decided to have her areola and nipple rebuilt. To obtain the nipple prominence, tissue from Pam's earlobe was used. The small, wedge-shaped piece removed from the earlobe left that earlobe virtually unaffected. The areola was simulated by using skin taken from the inner thigh area.

a normal woman. I guess you'd say I never accepted the idea of having one breast.

"I know it's not for every woman, but for me, it's something that has a certain importance and no matter what I tell myself, it won't change. I just feel I must have two breasts."

Frequently Asked Questions

Will reconstruction cause scars?

Any incision into tissue creates a scar. A plastic surgeon making incisions into tissue attempts to minimize scar formation but cannot eliminate it completely. The amount of scarring you will have from any reconstruction depends greatly on your specific circumstance. At times, the reconstruction may use previously placed mastectomy scars as a point of incision. The original scar may in fact be improved by reconstructive surgery. If a flap technique is used to transfer tissue, more scarring is necessary. The extent of the scar will improve with time, but some remnant will always remain. This is an important concern for some patients, especially when considering moving tissue from another area where a scar will remain.

How will I look after my reconstruction?

Results of reconstruction will vary depending on the scope of your mastectomy surgery and on your capacity to heal after surgery. The condition of the chest wall may vary. In the ideal situation where there is adequate skin overlying intact chest muscles, the results are generally excellent. Some women may have very thin, tight skin covering a chest wall where the underlying pectoral muscles have been removed. If radiation therapy has been done, some tissue in the area of the mastectomy may have been damaged. Your results will depend on these combinations of variable factors. In most situations, the reconstructed breast will look normal when it is covered with an undergarment. Uncovered, it will show some scarring and subtle imperfections. You should ask your plastic surgeon to show you pre- and postoperative photographs of different patients so you will have a better idea of your own potential postoperative looks.

Will my breasts match?

Most women's breasts do not match perfectly. Your new breast should be similarly proportioned to the other one and positioned symmetrically. Your surgeon will try to match your other breast, even if additional skin or muscle needs to be added to the mastectomy side. A breast uplift will help you achieve symmetry if the natural breast sags. If your natural breast is small and flattened, a breast implant can be used to enlarge it. If the natural breast is very large, it can be reduced in size and reshaped so it resembles the reconstructed breast.

How many procedures are necessary?

This depends on many factors. The extent of your mastectomy is one; how extensive you wish the reconstruction to be is another. Some patients want only the breast mound reconstructed because in a dress or bathing suit they appear normal. Many others want the mound rebuilt as well as having the nipple and areola reconstructed. In such a case you may need two or three separate procedures. However, the rebuilding of the nipple and areola are not complicated procedures and may be done in the surgeon's office.

I've heard that breast reconstruction can prevent the detection of a recurrence of my cancer. Is this true?

If a cancer recurs locally, it usually does so in the region of the mastectomy, in the skin. The implant is beneath the skin and, often, beneath the chest muscles. The reconstruction will not prevent your physician from detecting any recurring cancer. There is no evidence that breast reconstruction worsens the course of breast cancer. Certain reconstructive procedures may, in your case, not be reasonable because of the possibility of interfering with your follow-up care. This is an individual situation and must be discussed with your surgeon.

Will my breasts feel normal after my reconstruction?

Most reconstructed breasts are firmer than natural breasts, although some women have very soft and natural-feeling breasts after reconstruction. Rebuilding cannot restore normal sensation to a breast after mastectomy. If the nipple and areola are reconstructed, they do not retain normal sensation either.

Will I be able to wear a low neckline?

You may wear any kind of garment you wish. Most women have their breasts rebuilt for just such a purpose. How low a neckline you will want to wear will depend on the fullness of the upper half of your reconstructed breast. If scars remain from your mastectomy, these might be noticeable in certain clothes. It is best to talk with your general surgeon and plastic surgeon before the mastectomy about the positioning of the scars.

How long will I have to stay in the hospital?

This varies on the timing and kind of procedure you have. If reconstruction is combined with a mastectomy, it will not add any time to your hospital stay. If done separately with tissue expansion techniques, you may be discharged the morning after surgery. If extensive skin and muscle flaps are needed from donor sites elsewhere on your body, your hospital stay may be longer.

Can a breast reconstruction cause cancer?

There is no evidence that breast reconstruction will increase or decrease your chances of developing cancer. There is no evidence that it will cause a recurrence of a cancer that has been removed.

Can I sleep on my stomach after I have my breast rebuilt?

Most women agree that it takes a while to get used to having a reconstructed breast. After a while, when you have become accustomed to the new breast, you may rest in any position you wish.

After my reconstruction, what kind of follow-up care is needed?

You should have follow-up examinations by your plastic surgeon. At these visits the surgeon will make certain your implant (if used in the reconstruction) is in good condition and that the overlying skin is healthy. Your plastic surgeon will check for recurrences but you must see your general surgeon for your lifelong follow-up. This applies whether or not you have had a breast reconstructed. You must also remember to do regular BSE in *both* your reconstructed breast and the natural breast. This is necessary because no matter how thorough your surgeon was during your mastectomy or lumpectomy, usually some breast tissue cells remain behind. There is always the possibility such cells may become malignant.

ELEVEN

Life Beyond
Breast Cancer

❦

There *is* life beyond breast cancer. Hopefully, with advances in all areas of diagnosing and treating this disease, more and more women will live well beyond the point in their lives when breast cancer became a reality.

For any woman who has battled breast cancer there is the uncertainty of not knowing how long she will live. This will color her sense of herself, her future, and her life. How this affects the quality of her life depends, of course, on many things: her past experiences, her capacity to cope, her family, her friends, her career opportunities, and her other emotional resources.

The most telling words describing how different women deal with their lives after breast cancer were spoken by patients themselves.

❦ Pam Reimer continued with her life very much as before.
"It's been more than a year now, and I have a better idea of where I've been," said Pam after the successful

reconstruction of her breast. "I guess the thing I notice most now is that I'm much calmer than I used to be. I don't sweat the small stuff.

"When something goes wrong at the office, when we're behind and there's lots of briefs to catch up on, I don't go crazy the way I used to. And I think I'm different with people—I don't let little things annoy me the way they used to. I don't let people's pettiness or their little squabbles get to me. After what I've been through, I don't have time for that. There's too much out there that's precious to me and I just can't be bothered."

As for her breast reconstruction, Pam feels it was partly responsible for the way she now feels about her life.

"I feel great about it. The results were better than anything I could have hoped for. It was important to me, and it makes me feel like in some ways, I beat cancer.

"It's funny when I think about the changes I went through with this thing, I mean *real* changes. It made me think about things I never dreamed I'd think about—my life, dying, my relationships, what was important to me.

"I've thought about my sisters and my mother. And I think I understand us all a lot better than I ever did. I *really* do, now . . . and that was without a shrink [she laughs]. I know where they're coming from and how I always felt they got more than I did and how jealous I was. All of it . . . how we each had our problems . . . but you know what? It doesn't seem to matter very much anymore. I guess you'd say I'm more philosophical.

"John and I are much closer than we ever were. And like I said, I've got no doubts about him now. No doubts about *us*. We're really a team. And maybe it's because of the cancer—maybe it's because we know that we don't have

forever—but we do more than we used to do. This winter
we're going to the Caribbean and then we're thinking about
Mexico, and other trips.

"Sure, I think about the possibility that I might die. Doesn't
everyone? Maybe it's closer for me, or it could be years
and years away. But I'll tell you, I'm not going to worry
about it. I've got my husband and my son and my life to
live. My life's good, very good . . . better than I ever thought
it could be after breast cancer.

"When you really think about it, how long does anybody
have? And who knows what's down the line? I can't let it
worry me now. That's past me. And if something happens
in a few years, I'll take it from there [She laughs again].
Listen to me . . . a real hero!"

Pam's husband, John, reflected back on the time since
the diagnosis of Pam's breast cancer and how certain things
have changed.

"There's no question we've gotten closer since this all
began. We went through a traumatic time and we came
out winners!

"I'll tell you, one of the biggest things is the way I see
Pam differently now. In all honesty, if you'd asked me a
couple of years ago if I thought she could have gone through
a thing like this, if she'd be able to stand up to it the way
she has, I'd have said 'no.' The truth is I always thought
she was kind of a crybaby. But not now. I think it brought
something out in her. I admire her strength now . . . much
more than before.

"Sure, I worry sometimes that it might come back. And
I know I've been sensitized. If anything goes wrong—if she
gets a sniffle, a cough, any little thing—it makes me think
about the cancer. But that's the way I am.

"I got involved with her whole treatment. I mean, I did

things I never thought *I* could do. I read about breast cancer, I learned about this test and that one . . . got to be an 'expert.' And I questioned the doctors. I never thought I could do that. I forced myself to do it because I know that in a way I wanted to close my eyes and not get involved, not look at what was going on. But something inside me took over and I got more involved in Pam's treatment than she was.

"I'm different now, different in a better way. So is Pam. *We're* different. We've grown together because of what happened and I like the way we've changed."

❧ Unfortunately, not every patient adapts as well as Pam did. Janet McGovern was 42 when she developed a malignant mass in her left breast. The lesion was small and was detected early. No lymph nodes were involved. She had a lumpectomy with follow-up radiation.

One year later, she noticed a lump in her right breast, and, horrified, she promptly sought treatment. The lump was malignant, and three lymph nodes in the right axilla were involved. She had another lumpectomy and the lymph nodes were excised. She also had chemotherapy for 7 months.

The time during her chemotherapy was very difficult for Janet. She felt nauseated and weak and was despairing at the loss of her hair. Reassurances that this was temporary were not helpful. She became very depressed and was unable to do minimal work around the house. She became tearful and obsessed with morbid thoughts about death. Her husband and two teen-aged children helped all they could and tried to bolster her up, but to no avail.

When her chemotherapy was completed, her family thought Janet's spirits would improve, but she was as depressed as before. She feared she had metastatic disease and was convinced she would die in a year or two. She lost interest in all activities and had recurrent nightmares about her treatments, fearing she would have another recurrence and would need more chemotherapy.

Janet had been a bright and energetic wife and mother, but she was now listless, depressed, and pessimistic. She felt she had nothing to live for and was waiting to die. She became irritable with her family and spent days at a time in the bedroom, refusing to participate in any household or family activities.

Only after endless coaxing by her husband did she consent to have a follow-up examination. One year later, she was found to be free of signs of cancer. This seemed to raise her spirits slightly, and she began taking a minimal interest in her house and family during the next few months.

Nearly a year later she was still free of cancer but was still depressed. Finally, her husband convinced her to accompany him to a psychiatrist for counseling.

It is now 4 years since Janet McGovern's initial diagnosis of breast cancer. Although she is still symptom-free, she has not fully accommodated to her situation and is still convinced she will have another recurrence. Her psychotherapy sessions with her husband are filled with recriminations, and it is clear that problems that existed before the breast cancer have surfaced and are now taking their toll. Although Janet has made progress since her first session, she still has a way to go.

❧ Barbara Conti reflected back on her life after breast cancer.

"I still have this battle in my mind. On the one hand I tell myself, 'You're cured. It's been 12 years and you're cured.' But I still think about the possibility of a recurrence. I suppose that will never go away. I just hope I'm around to worry about it 30 years from now!

"I've come a long way in these 12 years. It sometimes seems to me that everything's changed . . . for the better. Don't get me wrong—I don't have any illusions about it. I wish I'd never had the cancer, but I *did.* You see, I just said *did,* using the past tense, which is wrong. I suppose I should say I *have* cancer, but it doesn't really matter. *Had* it or *have* it, it changed my life.

"In some ways, when I think about the reconstruction now, 12 years later, I guess I'm trying to get rid of the last bit of evidence of the cancer, and it took me all this time to feel comfortable about doing it. I never did adjust to having one breast . . . never. But I don't think I'm pretending anything away by having reconstruction now. The breast cancer will always be with me. If nothing else, it's in my mind.

"I'd have been better off without it, but I never had that choice. Just like I never chose the color of my hair or my height or my parents and their parents. I suppose I was lucky because it was diagnosed early, and so far, there's no evidence of recurrence or metastasis.

"It made me appreciate my life. Value it; be scared for it; other things too. My husband and I went through it together and it changed us, for the better. We grew closer because of it, but we each became a little more independent too, in some ways. I think that's because we had to suddenly imagine what life would be like without each other— especially Ted—because the reality was, I might die first. Neither of us had ever thought about that. Having cancer or any serious disease can do that, can make you think about things from another perspective. It makes you grow.

"About the independence—I'd taught school for years just

to have something to do. We were well off, and it was something to do. But after the cancer, it became important for me to push for something else, something that would be mine. That was the other side of the coin. As close as Ted and I became, we each grew a little in the other direction too, toward self-sufficiency. I'm going to be a school principal one of these days. I just know it."

Barbara's husband, Ted, was interviewed separately some months later. A corporation executive, he was a quiet and forceful man who spoke candidly about his life with Barbara.

"The shock of it all was incredible when it first happened, but it wears off. In the long run, it affected us very deeply.

"Barbara and I didn't want children. That was a decision we made years ago, long before her breast cancer. It didn't fit into the kind of life we wanted. After she was treated for the cancer, I found myself thinking about children, about how we'd made this decision which was pretty much irreversible. I began regretting it, that we didn't have children. I don't know if I wanted children so there'd be something of us both, something that would outlive us, or if I was worrying about the possibility that Barbara might die. That if she did, I'd be alone. That sounds pretty selfish, doesn't it?

"But cancer makes you think of things like that. How will I live without her? You try and imagine yourself alone, after all those years. Anyone who doesn't admit to having those thoughts isn't telling the truth.

"Barbara's breast cancer really tested us both because I suddenly discovered how scared I was at the thought I might lose her. And then, when she decided to *really* make a career out of the teaching—to become an assistant principal, and now a principal—with the meetings and the pressures, it made me wonder if we were drifting apart. She became

---

very involved with her work and needed something more in her life. I felt left out and frightened. I discovered that I was childish in some ways, and that sometimes I could be pretty selfish.

"But we kept at it and we've done all right. It's been twelve years and we've come a long way. Together . . . and individually."

❧ Three years after Lucille Greene was treated for breast cancer, she was actively taking courses in real estate and planned to take an examination for licensing as a realty broker.

"They were terrible times," Lucille said, reflecting back on her treatment. She had just been to her physician's office, where she went for her regular examination that included blood tests, a urinalysis, and a physical examination.

"I think the worst time was when I found the lump and had to wait for the diagnosis. Then, after the surgery . . . the chemotherapy. But it saved my life.

"Maybe it sounds corny but it was a learning experience . . . the whole thing. Bob and I discovered a lot about ourselves, and about each other.

"I'm a lot more confident about things now. I do things I never thought I could do. After what I've been through, anything seems easy.

"We're in counseling now because of how my illness affected Bob—how all the loving, tender feelings were there but he couldn't get back the sexy ones. I've learned that he's a much more complicated man than I ever thought. It really affected him—the way he sees me, himself, the kids. And we're trying to get things back on track. It's been an eye opener because things come up in the sessions that have nothing to do with the reasons we came in the first place, that have nothing to do with cancer. Things I wouldn't dream we'd be discussing together, or with someone else. It's opened us up to ourselves and to each other. And it's made us aware of problems that were there *before* I got sick. It's just that we weren't looking at them then.

"It's been rough on the kids, especially on Jean [her daughter]. It's hard being a young woman and not knowing if your mother will be alive in a few years. But that's what she has to cope with. It's what we all have to cope with. And Jean, she's in the high-risk group now. I know that bothers her.

"But I think we'll do fine, all of us. Because you have to move on. You have to deal with the unknown, and with things that aren't always nice. You have to deal with each thing as it comes up, with the changes in your life, one by one. You learn to be flexible, to cope. And you never know. That's life."

· *TWELVE* ·

The Future

Some time from now, much of this book will be obsolete. Enormous strides will have been made in understanding breast cancer, its early diagnosis, and its treatment. This will probably occur for all cancers. Progress seems likely to be most dramatic in understanding the basic mechanisms of the disease process and in its treatment. There may even be major steps made toward the prevention of breast cancer. In this chapter, we will speculate about the advances we think will most probably be made within the next few years.

Advances in Understanding the Disease

A host of crucial questions must be answered and understood before scientists and physicians have a full understanding of breast cancer and of cancers in general. Right now, intensive investigations are underway in many areas of cellular biology and genetics so that certain practical solutions may emerge in the early detection and treatment of breast cancer.

For instance, what are the stresses or other factors that

cause a cell to begin replicating in an uncontrollable manner? Ordinarily, normal tissues are capable of speeding up and then slowing down the process of duplication in an appropriate way. If you injure your skin, there is a sudden "speeding up" of the process of cellular duplication to about forty times the normal rate. In this way, the skin repairs itself and continues to function normally. At the appropriate time, when the injury is repaired, cell division slows down and proceeds at its normal rate. How does the cell manage to "know" when to speed up and slow down without departing from its normal reproductive cycle? What are the modifiers of cell replication, and how do they work? Why and how have they stopped working properly in the disease state called cancer?

When an embryo first forms, over the course of a few weeks, cell replication proceeds at a very rapid rate. From a one-celled organism, the embryo proceeds to divide and subdivide over the course of weeks into an organism composed of millions of cells. This, of course, is normal. Then, at an appropriate time, this process of cell replication slows down. How and why? What modifying influences are at work here? Is the cancer cell in some way returning to this earlier, embryonic state of functioning?

Why do these cellular changes occur in some tissues such as the breast, the lung, or the colon? Is the process of cancer formation in the breast the same as that of the colon? Of the lung? All these questions and many more are under investigation even as you read these words. We can only hope right now that research scientists are very close to achieving a better understanding of the structure and function of genetic substances such as DNA and RNA, which will lead to dramatic advances in the prevention, screening, diagnosis, and treatment of breast cancer.

Advances in Prevention

Since prevention of any disease is preferable to treatment, we hope this area will yield dramatic advances. Here are two developments with promise:

Diet may play a more important role in the development of breast cancer than has been generally acknowledged. Researchers now have epidemiologic evidence that women whose dietary intake of fat is decreased and who eat more fiber have a lower incidence of breast cancer than other women. In our view, diet alone is probably not the entire answer, but certain women may enhance their chances of preventing breast cancer by adhering to a low-fat, high-fiber diet. This approach certainly merits further study.

An *oncogene* (cancer gene) has been discovered to play a role in the formation of certain cancers. If such a gene can be isolated and studied, certain anti-oncogene factors may be discovered or synthesized. Conceivably, such an anti-cancer substance could be used prophylactically to prevent not only breast cancer, but all cancers.

Advances in Screening

Right now, *breast self-examination* is the least expensive routine screening procedure available to the most women. The more information about BSE that is disseminated to the general public, the more aware women will be about its importance. This could lead to earlier reporting of suspicious signs or symptoms of the disease. Statistics show that when such detection and reporting methods are consistently used, the death rate from breast cancer drops dramatically.

We have already mentioned *CAT screen mammography,* which may become more readily available as the financial cost of sophisticated technology is reduced. The special characteristics of this technique allow the physician to obtain a very sensitive illustration of even the smallest tumor mass. It offers the physician special information about any breast mass and is very important when evaluating patients who have severe fibrocystic disease of the breast, where ordinary mammograpy is of limited use.

Nuclear Magnetic Resonance (NMR) is the latest and promises to be the most revolutionary detection method. This technique is non-invasive and does not use any form of radiation. A magnetic field is formed around the patient's body, and computer analysis allows for a visual representation of the internal workings of the body. The picture produced depends on the fact that various body tissues and cells interact differently with the electromagnetic field.

This technique is capable of highlighting even the most minute differences between normal and abnormal tissues. As can be done with CAT screen mammography, a pictorial representation can be made of various levels of the tissue under examination, much like slicing a loaf of bread. This technique will revolutionize cancer detection and many other areas of medicine as well. It will be the most powerful diagnostic tool physicians have ever had.

At present, NMR is being used in a few pilot programs and is not yet available as a detection tool. It will take more time and investigation to lower the very high cost of NMR before it is found in most hospital centers.

Tumor markers have been discovered in certain types of cancers. A tumor marker is a substance produced by cancerous cells and is found in the tissues of patients who have that kind of cancer. The quest for such a specific biochemical indicator means determining the nature of the substance released by the tumor and also developing equipment sensitive enough to detect it in the smallest concentrations. This substance is released into the body tissues and bloodstream as the tumor begins its growth. This marker could then be detected by a routine blood test at the earliest possible time. Then, even before the disease manifests itself, appropriate treatment may be undertaken. In theory, as the tumor is treated, the amount of biochemical marker will decrease. This can be measured quantitatively and provides a basis for assessing the patient's progress.

Advances in Treatment

Within the realm of the currently foreseeable, we anticipate the following progress in the treatment of breast cancers:
Immunotherapy may soon become a reality. It has been maintained that in patients who develop cancer, there is a decrease in immunologic competence. Simply put, the body's natural defense mechanisms seem to be decreased in patients with breast cancer. It has also been demonstrated that these defense mechanisms become further depressed as a tumor grows and increases in size.

We know that along with the primary tumor, there are often malignant changes present either in that breast or in the other breast. After the primary tumor is removed, some of these small aggregates of tumor cells may progress to life-threatening tumors while others revert to normal. Could it be that sometimes, when the tumor is removed, the patient's immune system is then capable of destroying these small aggregates of malignant cells? All this is under intensive investigation.

Research scientists are trying to determine how the immune system may be stimulated to respond normally in the face of cancer cells or even be stimulated to overrespond, manufacturing a variety of substances that would seek out and destroy invading cancer cells. This has long been done with bacteria and viruses where various toxoids are given to stimulate the body's production of antitoxins.

Surgery has become more refined, and today, increasing numbers of women who are at high risk for developing breast cancer are choosing to have prophylactic subcutaneous mastectomies. This is an aggressive approach and is somewhat controversial, but for certain high-risk women it has proven to be very useful. Now that reconstructive techniques providing excellent results are available, this avenue of attack may help stem the tide until the basic disease process is better understood. Then, breast cancer can be treated by other means or even prevented.

This raises another issue. Some patients have asked if subcutaneous mastectomy is a reasonable treatment choice for women who have small, local breast cancers. Such an approach would, of course, eliminate the disfiguring aspect of breast surgery.

At this time, subcutaneous mastectomy is not done to treat breast cancer because there are not yet any long-term studies of treatment results. But this may very well be another surgical option for future patients. More and more prophylactic subcutaneous mastectomies are being done. Postsurgical microscopic examination of the removed breast tissue reveals that a percentage of these patients were harboring undetected cancers. Therefore, as time passes, an increasing number of women will, practically speaking, have been treated for breast cancer by this method. Over time, doctors will be able to determine the rate of recurrence or metastasis in this growing population of patients. The statistical results that emerge will reveal whether subcutaneous mastectomy may be a reasonable treatment option for certain breast cancers.

Radiation may play an increasing role in combating breast cancer. As we study more about the multifocal nature of breast cancers, radiation techniques may continue to improve and become even more effective. If targeting of radiation could be greatly improved, it may eventually be used to treat small multifocal areas of cancer without affecting the surrounding normal tissue.

Chemotherapy will no doubt become a more effective treatment tool for patients in whom the disease has spread beyond the breast. There is presently a search for chemotherapy agents that will deal directly with cancer cells. Such agents will be more *tumor-specific;* that is, they will attack and destroy cancer cells while bypassing the body's normal cells. This would mean effective chemotherapy with very few side effects.

Just as bacteria can be cultured in the laboratory, it may soon be possible to remove one or two cancer cells from a tumor, culture them in a laboratory, and then test their sensitivity to various cancer-killing drugs. Then the specific drug for that particular type of cancer cell may be used in a course of chemotherapy.

Genetic engineering may be a means to eventually combat cancer of all types. It is conceivable that the genetic code by which all cells (including cancerous ones) reproduce may be entirely cracked. Then, physicians may be able to interrupt the cycle of cancer cell proliferation, even before a tumor forms. This would mean first learning the coding sequence of various cells' reproductive cycles and, of course, depends on science's eventually developing a better understanding of the basic disease process.

Within the medical profession, we hope the myopic and self-serving controversies concerning the "best" treatment for breast cancer may soon come to an end. Hopefully, physicians will realize that only by a team approach with the sharing of new insights and innovative techniques among specialists will patients be most helped to deal with breast cancer.

The future is very bright. Most likely, basic research and clinical medicine will merge their findings, ushering in a new era in the understanding and treatment of breast cancer. Your daughter and her daughter will probably have a very different perspective on this disease.

At this moment, however, we must face the undeniable reality that the major hope for battling breast cancer is through early detection by so simple a method as breast self-examination, followed by prompt diagnosis and treatment of any suspicious breast change. This means that every woman must be knowledgeable about her own body. Above all, it means every woman must be responsible for her health and be willing to play an active role in learning her treatment choices and maintaining her own well-being.

Index

Boldface page numbers indicate material in illustrations.

Abortion, 23–24
Age of woman
 older women, 75, 163
 and risk of cancer, 11, 22
Anesthesia, 121, 123–24
Anger, 60, 74, 75–76, 78, 126, 128
 of husband, 80
Areola
 banking, 179
 rebuilding, 177–79
Armpit
 lymph nodes in, 5, **6**
 swelling of, 28–29
Attractiveness, woman's sense of, 60–
 61, 71–74, 128

Benign lumps and tumors, ix, 3. *See
 also* Fibrocystic disease.
 percentage of, 7, 26, 30
Bias of physicians, 91, 101–3, 104
Biopsy, 51–55
Breast
 anatomy of, 4, **5**
 changes in tissue of, 6–7, 36
 opposite, treatment of, 110–13, 180
 pain in, 29
 swelling or dimpling of, 28
Breast Pap test, 47
Breast self-examination (BSE), 30–38
 as early-detection strategy, 19, 30–31,
 201, 206
 failure to practice, reasons for, 31–
 34
 in pregnancy, 46

Cancer
 development of, 2–3, 7–9
 genetic component of, 2. *See also*
 Family history of cancer.
 invasive, 8
 metastasized. *See* Metastasis.
 secondary, 4, 56, 89, 114–15, 117
Cancer Information Clearinghouse,
 133
Cancerphobia, 83–84
CAT scan mammography, 45, 201–2
Causes of breast cancer
 misconceptions about, 10–11
 stress as, 22–23, 199–200
 virus as, 23
Cell reproduction, 1–2
Chemotherapy, 115–18, 205
 coping with, 135–37
 with lumpectomy, 95
 side effects of, 97, 115, 116–17
Childbearing history, 14, 23
Children, informing about mother's illness, 79, 158–59
Cigarette smoking, 24
Clothing, 163–64, 167, 188
Communication
 with doctor, 62–64
 with family, 140–41
 with hospital staff, 122
 with husband, 149–50, 154, 157
Contraceptives, oral, 15
Control, patient's, 54, 168. *See also*
 Treatment: deciding on.

Counseling, psychological, 81, 84, 112, 129, 131
   for depression, 82, 129, 147, 194
Cure of breast cancer, 143
   and early detection, 30, 34, 90, 206
   and lumpectomy-radiation treatment, 101
   and lymph-node involvement, 89–90
   and radical mastectomy, 93
Cysts. See Benign lumps and tumors; Fibrocystic disease, benign; Tumor(s).

Daughter(s) of women with breast cancer, 77, 159, 198. See also Family history of cancer.
Death and dying
   attitude toward, 61, 68, 78–79, 126, 192
   "inevitability" of (myth of), 78, 87, 140, 153, 162–63
Deformity and mutilation, 33, 71, 78, 130
   men and, 151
Denial, 33, 77, 82–83, 126, 140, 169–70
Depression, 65–66, 78, 81–82, 145–48, 194
   chemotherapy and, 117
   mastectomy and, 129–30
DES (diethylstilbestrol), 14–15
Detection of breast cancer, 26–48, 101–3
   early, importance of, 19, 26, 30–31, 34, 90, 206
   by self-examination. See Breast self-examination (BSE).
   See also Mammography; Nuclear Magnetic Resonance; Thermography; Ultrasound.
Diagnosis, 49–66
   interval following, before treatment, 53, 54–55, 58, 64, 78, 104
   responses to, 56–61, 67–85. See also Biopsy; Tests.

Diet, 15–16, 201
Doctor(s)
   bias of, 91, 101–3, 104
   referrals of, 104, 105, 109, 147
   relationship with patient, 61–64, 66
   selection of, 49
   teamwork of, 86, 87, 103–5
Drug therapy. See Chemotherapy.

Emotions. See Feelings and emotions.
Endocrine therapy, 118
Environmental influences, 3
Estrogen
   replacement therapy, 20, 24
   and risk of cancer, 14–15
   tumors dependent on, 55–56, 118
Ethnic origin, as risk factor, 17
Exercise, and cancer, 24–25

Family history of cancer, 2, 21
Family of cancer patient
   communication with, 140–41
   impact of cancer on, 70, 139–40
   support from, 79, 124–25, 131, 141, 147.
   See also Children; Husband(s); Marriage.
Fatal, cancer as (myth of), 78, 87, 140, 153, 162–63
Fear
   of anesthesia, 121
   of breast cancer, ix, 27, 56–58, 61, 68–71, 78
   and BSE, 32, 33
   of death, 61, 68, 78–79, 126, 192
   of deformity, mutilation, 33
Feelings and emotions
   acceptance of, 123
   anger, 60, 74, 75–76, 78, 126, 128
   failure, sense of, 69
   guilt, 60, 76–77, 140
   of husband, 80, 82, 148–58, 192–93, 196–97
   impact of, on treatment decision, 99–100

in response to diagnosis of cancer,
  56–61, 67–85.
  See also Fear.
Fibrocystic disease, benign, 7, 26
  pain as sign of, 29
  and risk of cancer, 12, 14
  ultrasound detection of, 43
Follow-up, medical, 137–38, 189

Genetic component of cancer, 2. *See
  also* Family history of cancer.
Genetic engineering, 205
Groups, self-help, 131–33, 153
Growth rate of tumors, 7–9
Guilt, 60, 76–77, 140

Halsted radical mastectomy, 92–93
Health insurance, 104, 160, 168
Hereditary component of cancer. *See*
  Family history of cancer.
High-risk women, 20. *See also* Family
  history of cancer.
  anxiety of, 83–84
  and incidence of cancer, 17
  mammography for, 42–43
  strategies for, 19–20
  and subcutaneous mastectomy, 112–
    13
Hormonal therapy, 118
Hormone-receptor assay, 55–56, 118
Hormones
  and risk of cancer, 14–15.
  See also Estrogen; Progesterone.
Hospitalization, 120–25, 188
Husband(s). *See also* Family of cancer
  patient.
  informing about wife's cancer, 79–80
  relationship with, 145–58, 191–93,
    195–97. *See also* Sexuality.
  responses of, to wife's cancer, 80, 82,
    148–58, 192–93, 196–97
Hypochondria, 33, 130, 142

Immune system
  and goal-setting, 144
  and metastasis, 89

stress and, 23
  weakened, signs of, 21
Immunotherapy, 203–4
Implant(s), for radiotherapy, 96
Implant(s), silicone
  and risk of cancer, 20–21
  in subcutaneous mastectomy, 111–
    13
"Inevitability" of death from cancer
  (myth of), 78, 87, 140, 153, 162–
    63
Insurance, 104, 160, 168
Interval between diagnosis and treat-
  ment, 53, 54–55, 58, 64, 78, 104
Invasive cancer, 8

Jobs and work life, 159–63

Law on informing cancer patients of options, 102–3
Life after breast cancer, 190–98
Loss of breast
  adjustment to, 125–26, 128, 130–31
  feelings about, 59, 61, 69, 71–75, 149
  men and, 148–58
Lumpectomy (tylectomy)
  with radiotherapy, 94–95
  survival rates for, 101
Lump(s) in breast. *See also* Tumor(s).
  benign, percentage of, 7, 26, 30
  detection of, 26–48
  painfulness of, 29, 38
  size of, 7
  as symptom of cancer, 28–29
  time needed for development of, 7–
    8
Lymphatic system, 4–6, **6**, 8, 89
Lymph nodes, 5, **6**, 89–90, 114
  surgical removal of, 98

Mammography, 38–43, 51
  computerized, tomographic, 45–46,
    201–2
  and metastasis, 88
  radiation risk from, 40–41, 48

Marriage. *See also* Husband(s).
  cancer as threat to, 151–52, 157–58, 197–98
  communication in, 149–50, 154, 157
Mastectomy
  and depression, 129
  feelings about, 108–9, 125–31
  men's response to, 148, 150
  modified radical, 93, **127**
  partial, 94
  radical, 92–93
  scars from, 126, **127,** 148–49
  second opinion on, 55
  subcutaneous, 111–13, 180, 182, 204
Medical insurance, 104, 160, 168
Men. *See also* Husband(s).
  breast cancer in, 21
  response of, to mastectomy, 148, 150
  telling about cancer, 155–56
Menstrual history, 14, 146–47
Metastasis, 3–4, 9
  and hormone dependency, 56
  testing for, 54, 88–89
  and treatment strategy, 86, 114, 117
Misconceptions and myths
  about causes of cancer, 10–11
  doctor and, 63
  about "inevitability" of death from cancer, 78, 87, 140, 153, 162–63
  about radiotherapy, 134
  about workers who had cancer, 160
Mitosis, 2
Mutilation. *See* Deformity and mutilation.

Needle biopsy, 51–52
Nipple(s)
  banking, 179
  discharge from, 29, 51
  inverted, 21, 28
  irritation of, 29
  rebuilding, 177–78, 179
Nuclear Magnetic Resonance (NMR), 202

Older women, 75, 163
Opposite breast, treatment of, 110–13, 180

Paget's disease, 29
Pain, 29, 38
Physician(s). *See* Doctor(s).
Prediction of cancer, 10, 17
Progesterone, 55–56, 118
Prosthesis
  external, 167
  silicone, 176
Psychiatric counseling. *See* Counseling, psychological.

Radiation. *See also* Radiotherapy.
  from mammography, 40–41, 48
  and risk of cancer, 16–17
Radical mastectomy, 92–93
  modified, 93, **127**
Radiotherapy, 95–98, 205
  combined with surgery, 93–95
  controversy over, 91
  coping with, 133–35
  implant of, 96
  side effects of, 97, 98
Reach to Recovery program, 131–32
Reconstruction of breast, 165–89, **183–85**
  candidates for, 169–71
  complications from, 176–77
  as hope for breast cancer patients, 59, 70, 72, 107, 128–29, 151, 156, 191, 195
  older women and, 75
  and opposite breast, 111, 180
  postoperative period, 181–82, 186
  reasons for reluctance about, 75, 163
  techniques of, 173–79
  timing of, 171–73
Recurrence of cancer
  detection of, after reconstruction, 187–88
  fear of, 61, 69–70, 130, 141–45, 146, 194–95

after radical mastectomy, 93.
See also Cure of breast cancer.
Referral of doctors, 104, 105, 109, 147
Risk factors, 11–19

Scars, 126, **127,** 148–49, 166–67,
183–85, 186
Secondary tumor(s), 4, 56, 89, 114–15,
117. *See also* Metastasis.
Second opinion, 54, 55, 104
Self-examination. *See* Breast self-exam-
ination (BSE).
Self-help groups, 131–33, 153
Self-image and self-esteem, 60–61, 71–
74, 128, 163, 167
Sexuality, breast cancer as threat to, 60,
73, 128, 145–58
Side effects
of chemotherapy, 97, 115, 116–17,
136
of radiotherapy, 97, 98
Silicone implants
and risk of cancer, 20–21
in subcutaneous mastectomy, 111–
13
Single women, 148, 155–56
Size of lumps and tumors, 7, 105–6
Spreading of cancer cells. *See* Metastasis.
Stages of breast cancer, 90–91
Stress, as risk factor, 22–23, 199–200
Subcutaneous mastectomy, 111–13,
180, 182, 204
Surgical procedures
biopsy, 52–55
combined with radiotherapy, 93–95
controversy over, 91
mastectomy. *See* Mastectomy.
reconstruction. *See* Reconstruction
of breast.
Survival rates. *See* Cure of breast cancer.
Symptoms of breast cancer, 27–30

Tamoxifen™ (drug), 56, 118
Tests
Breast Pap test, 47
hormone-receptor assay, 55–56,
118
for malignancy (biopsy), 51–55
for metastasis, 54, 88–89
See also Diagnosis.
Thermography, 44–45
Transillumination of breast, 50
Treatment, 86–113, 203–6
deciding on, 86–87, 98–109
of local, regional disease, 91–98
of opposite breast, 110–13
options in, 55, 91, 98–101
systemic, 114–19
team approach to, 86, 87, 103–5.
See also Chemotherapy; Endocrine
therapy; Immunotherapy; Radiotherapy; Surgical procedures.
Tumor(s), 2, 3
benign, 3
growth rate of, 7–9
malignant, 3–4, 38
multifocal, 12
secondary, 4, 56, 89, 114–15, 117
size and location of, 7, 105–6.
See also Lump(s) in breast.
Tumor markers, 202–3
Tylectomy (lumpectomy), 94–95, 101

Ultrasound, 43–44
Uterus, cancer of, 21

Virus, as cause of cancer, 23

We the Victors, 143–44
White blood cells, 5, 89
Will to live, 125, 144
Work life, 159–63

X-rays. *See* Radiation; Radiotherapy.